HOW TO WRITE AN EXERCISE PROGRAM

A STEP-BY-STEP GUIDE TO BECOMING YOUR OWN PERSONAL TRAINER

BY JEZ BLACKMORE

Published by Urbacise Ltd

Company Number: 11248483

www.urbacise.com

ISBN Number: **978-1-9996064-0-4**

CONTENTS

GETTING THE SUPPORTING MEDIA

This book teaches you how to write your own exercise program, step-by-step. To keep this book from becoming needlessly complicated, we have put more detailed explanations of the technical concepts in the appendix at the back.

Supplementary information is also available on our website. The principles in this book are sound and deliver a solid foundation on which you can build, but the Urbacise website allows us to continuously add more value without having to republish.

For exercise articles, including advice on training, please visit: Urbacise.com/articles

Throughout this book you'll find links and references that highlight where you can find more information in the appendices and on our website. These include free resources such as templates, exercise logs, generic exercise programs and more.

To access our free templates, go to the download area of the website (free registration required): Urbacise.com/download/

This book also includes demonstrations on how to use exercises to target different muscle groups. For a more in-depth list of exercises, including example videos on how to perform each one, use our exercise database. This includes a filter feature, so you can effortlessly choose the correct exercises for you: Urbacise.com/exercises/

For extra support or to contribute to the Urbacise community, follow us on social media or get involved with the additional features Urbacise.com offers.

MOTIVATION FOR THIS BOOK

Before I became obsessed with working out, I remember how lost I felt when I visited a gym. I used to wander around looking at all the different exercise machines. They all seemed simple enough, but at the back of my mind I was asking myself, "Is this the best exercise for me?"

I didn't know the science behind any of these machines. Was I using them optimally? Should I be using them in a specific order? Should I be doing these exercises until failure? Which exercise would benefit my fitness goals the most?

With all these questions rattling around in my head, I hired a personal trainer. I paid hourly for each session, plus an extra fee for a four-week workout program. I exercised with my trainer twice a week and did his workout program in between sessions.

Working with a personal trainer was a great experience, and I saw my fitness level improve significantly. I began using the machines less and using free weights more. I learned the correct exercise form: how to lift weights and perform exercises correctly to reduce the risk of injury. However, I still didn't fully understand the techniques and science behind a workout program and was spending a lot of money each month.

After a while, I wondered if my trainer was just choosing random exercises and writing them down in a list, or if his approach was more scientific.

To save money, I stopped working with my personal trainer and began to educate myself about fitness and how the body reacts to working out. I learned how muscles tear under tension and grow back stronger, about the effects of cardio training, and the different techniques top personal trainers use to create a workout program. Being able to write a workout program myself would save me a lot of money, and I would also be exercising as efficiently as possible.

Now that I have all this information, I thought the next step would be to share my knowledge in the form of a book. I still see people wandering around the gym, not looking very confident or knowing what exercise to do next.

So here it is. This book aims to give you a guide to constructing your own workout programs. These won't be random lists of exercises, but well-structured and systematic plans to suit your fitness goals. You will save yourself money and start exercising with professional methodologies. With the knowledge and advice in this book, you'll know the secrets behind fitness and feel a lot more confident in the gym.

WHAT THIS BOOK WILL (AND WON'T) TEACH YOU

This book simply aims to educate you about exercise. Instead of selling you an exercise program, we provide the knowledge you need so you'll never have to buy an exercise program again! We do this by deconstructing the essential elements of an exercise program, looking at everything from basic anatomy to how long you should rest between sets.

The principles in this book can be adapted to suit all levels. If anything seems too complicated or difficult, you may not yet be at that level. For people who are relatively inexperienced in the gym or who prefer to work out at home, you can use these techniques for bodyweight or light resistance training.

You should use the advice and techniques in this book to individually customize your exercise programs based on your goals, experience, commitment level and how quickly your body recovers after a workout.

When speaking about exercise, there are four different types:

- **Aerobic**. Also known as cardio, these exercises strengthen your heart, lungs, and improve your body's overall efficiency in using oxygen. Normally consisting of exercises done over longer periods, such as brisk walks, distance running or road biking.

- **Anaerobic**. Is where you work at very high intensity or at your maximum level of exertion for a shorter period. These are typically exercises designed to improve strength, speed, and power, an example would be weight-lifting.
- **Flexibility**. These exercises improve the range of motion of your joints, allowing them to move freely and improve the overall mobility of your muscles.
- **Stability**. Without the correct alignment of your joints, you use your muscles to try to compensate. These exercises fix that problem.

This book mainly focuses on anaerobic and aerobic exercise, rather than flexibility and stability. We also only touch briefly on nutrition. To learn more about nutrition and other aspects of fitness you can visit Urbacise.com.

We aim to answer a lot of common questions about exercise so you can best structure your workout routines and train efficiently to meet your fitness goals quicker than you otherwise would. By the end of this book, you will have a much better understanding of the science behind exercise. Using professional methods, you will be able to structure your exercise programs or use your new expertise as a foundation towards a career in the fitness industry.

CHAPTER ONE: DEFINE YOUR GOALS

If you're reading this book, you are probably looking to learn about all the professional techniques used by fitness professionals, in order to write your own exercise programs and become more confident while exercising. But to start, it's always a good idea to ask yourself questions to better define your fitness goals. So, the first questions are: Do you want to:

- Lose fat?
- Gain muscle?
- Tone your body?
- Increase your strength?
- Become fitter?
- Get ready for a sporting event?
- Rehabilitate an injury?

The answer you choose will help decide your long-term goals, and thus your exercises and the frequency and intensity at which you train. It's important that your training goals are realistic and achievable, otherwise you might become disheartened and lose motivation.

Some other questions that will help make sure your long-term goal is realistic:

WHAT IS YOUR CURRENT BODY FAT PERCENTAGE?

If you want to look lean or achieve a certain aesthetic, your Body Fat Percentage (BFP) will play an important role. Having low body fat also generally means you're healthier overall. There's a limit, though: our bodies have "essential fats" that keep us warm and protect our organs and joints, so it's dangerous to have a body fat percentage below 5%. A healthy body fat percentage for men is 8% to 17% and for women it is 15% to 24%.

The table below shows the different body fat percentages for men and women. The easiest way to measure your body fat is to buy a "Skinfold Body Fat Caliper" or you could use body fat scales, available to buy online. There may even be one at your local fitness center.

	Men	**Women**
Essential Fats	2-5%	10-13%
Athletes	6-13%	14-20%
Fitness	14-17%	21-24%
Average	18-24%	25-31%
Obese	25%+	32%+

HOW MUCH FOOD DO YOU EAT?

The more food you eat, the more calories you're going to consume, and any unused calories will be stored in the body as glycogen or fat. In order to stay healthy, it is said, the average woman needs to consume around 2,000 calories each day and the average man around 2,500 calories (this figure can change based on your activity level). It's a good idea to educate yourself about the foods you eat or seek advice from a professional dietitian to calculate your ideal daily calorie intake.

HOW MANY UNITS OF ALCOHOL DO YOU DRINK EACH WEEK?

As we're all aware, drinking alcohol increases health risks. It's recommended that men and women should not drink more than 14 units of alcohol each week. The average pint of beer has 3 units, and the average glass of wine 2-3 units.

Alcohol also has a lot of calories. An average pint of beer has 180 calories, and a glass of wine has around 120 calories. To see quicker results through exercise you might want to consider cutting back on the alcohol. While we're at it, the same applies to full-fat fizzy drinks that contain a lot of calories.

HOW MUCH WATER DO YOU DRINK EVERY DAY?

There are many different opinions on how much water a person should be drinking each day. However, it's universally agreed that drinking water is good for you. Drinking water is especially important while exercising as it prevents you from dehydrating. The recommended water intake per day tends to be around two liters or half a gallon.

HOW MUCH SLEEP DO YOU GET EACH NIGHT?

Sleep is a critical time period for the body to recover and repair itself. Therefore, physicians recommend 8-10 hours of quality sleep per night. Adequate rest is also necessary for proper muscular growth. Without proper rest your body will not recover and you will not be able to reap the full benefits of your workout.

DO YOU HAVE ANY MEDICAL CONDITIONS OR INJURIES THAT MIGHT PREVENT YOU FROM DOING EXERCISE?

If you have any injuries or a medical condition that might prevent you from exercising, we strongly recommend you seek the advice of a medical professional before attempting any exercises or fitness activities.

WHAT IS THE TIME SPAN TO ACHIEVE YOUR FITNESS GOAL?

When I started on my fitness journey, I had no idea what was realistic, how long would it take me to lose a few pounds, or how strong would I be able to get in a month? The answers to these questions are determined by your commitment level and the discipline you show in your exercise activities and eating habits. However, there is an upper limit to what you'll be able to accomplish in a given time frame, based on your body's own biology. It's estimated, for example, that you need to burn around 3,500 calories to lose just 1 pound of fat. It's also estimated that the average person can only gain a maximum of between 2-3 pounds of muscle per month. Remember, when determining a timeframe to meet your fitness goals, keep it realistic. At first, it might not seem like you're making much progress. But over time, you'll be amazed by the results.

HOW FAMILIAR ARE YOU WITH PROPER FORM FOR USING FREE WEIGHTS?

If you have never used weights before and don't have the correct form when performing an exercise, it's very easy to injure yourself. We recommend you learn correct form before performing any weighted exercise. Form, in exercise, is based on your body's biomechanics and makes lifting a heavy load a lot safer.

WHAT'S YOUR CURRENT LEVEL OF STRENGTH/FITNESS?

To help decide if your goals are achievable and to help measure your progress, there are baseline fitness tests that we'll be discussing in the next chapter.

With your fitness goals, it's advisable to set long, medium and short-term goals. This will make sure you stay motivated.

When you tell a personal trainer your fitness goals, they will try to make sure they are achievable by using a principle called the "SMART" principle:

S – Specific: Keep your goals clear and simple.

M – Measurable: Track the progress to make sure you're achieving your goals.

A – Achievable: Is your goal unrealistic?

R – Relevant: Are you motivated to achieve your goals? Is your goal important to you?

T – Time-bound: Give yourself a deadline to meet your goal. This will help motivate you.

HOW MANY DAYS A WEEK ARE YOU GOING TO WORK OUT?

You should look at your schedule and determine the maximum amount of time and the specific days you will dedicate to exercising each week. This will help you later when determining how to structure your exercise program and split your workouts throughout the week. Don't worry about recovery for now. We'll address that a bit later. For now, just choose the maximum number of days you are willing to commit to fitness.

YOUR PROGRESS SHOULD BE MEASURABLE

As previously mentioned, at the start of your fitness journey, it's always a good idea to know your baseline fitness. That way, as you progress, you can compare yourself throughout your transformation and know that you're seeing improvement.

It's standard practice to measure your fitness progress by way of testing. Fitness testing, when done correctly, is one of the best ways to track your progress — unlike weight or Body Mass Index (BMI), which can sometimes be deceptive. Achieving a better result each time you perform a fitness test is more indicative of improvement than simply showing a lower BMI or a lower number on the scale. In fact, when it comes to your fitness level, your BMI and the number on your scale don't tell the whole story.

The main factors a personal trainer in the gym will test (if you had a consultation) will be your:

- Muscular Endurance
- Cardiovascular Fitness
- Strength
- Flexibility

Testing is measured through tables, where you can compare your results with others in your demographic, based on your age and gender.

The most popular fitness tests are:

- Crunch Test
- Push-up Test
- Three Minute Step Test
- Cooper Test
- Sergeant Jump Test
- Standing Long Jump Test
- Sit and Reach Test

MUSCULAR ENDURANCE TESTS

1. CRUNCH TEST

This test assesses your abdominal endurance. Please note that this is not the standard sit-up test. In fact, crunches are a lot better than full sit-ups because they are easier on your lower back. Furthermore, you will be able to engage and target your abdominals more than you would if you were doing sit-ups. This test is very simple because you can do it at home or at the gym, and all you will need is a stopwatch. The purpose of this test is to determine how many crunches, with proper form, you can do in one minute.

In order to perform the crunches, lie down flat on your back with your knees bent. Your feet should be flat on the floor. Your heels should be about 16-20 inches away from your butt. Place your arms flat at your sides so that your fingertips are near your hips. Measure and mark off six inches forward from your fingertips. Then, engage your abs to lift your head, neck and shoulder blades off the floor.

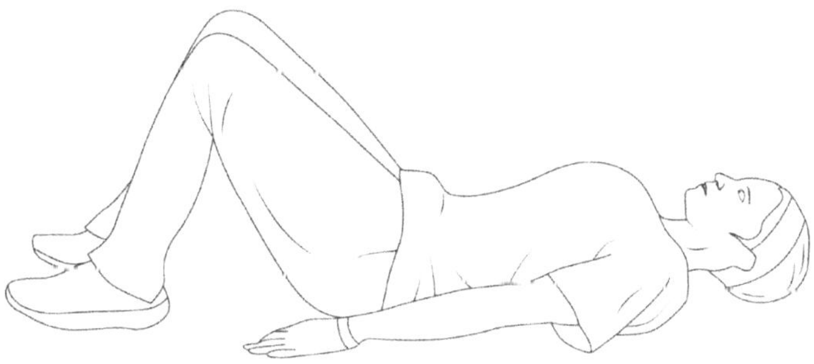

You should only count the reps where your fingertips surpass the six-inch marker.

Once the minute is up, it's time to analyze your results. To see where you stand, please look at the tables below based on your age and gender:

MEN

Rating	< 35 years	35-44 years	> 45 years
Excellent	60	50	40
Good	45	40	25
Marginal	30	25	15
Needs Work	15	10	5

WOMEN

Rating	< 35 years	35-44 years	> 45 years
Excellent	50	40	30
Good	40	25	15
Marginal	25	15	10
Needs Work	10	6	4

Figures based on guidelines published by the American College of Sports Medicine (ACSM)

2. PUSH-UP TEST

The push-up test is one of the best ways to measure your upper body endurance. It's a lot safer than the one-rep max for bench press, which is more about muscular strength than endurance. The push-up test can be done anytime and anywhere, if you have something that you can time yourself with. The purpose of this test is to see how many push-ups you can do in one minute, using proper form.

For the purpose of this test, women should perform a modified push-up version (on their knees). Men, on the other hand, must start with hands shoulder-width apart (on the floor) and be up on their toes. Both genders must keep their body as straight as possible, to avoid bending at the waist when performing the push-ups.

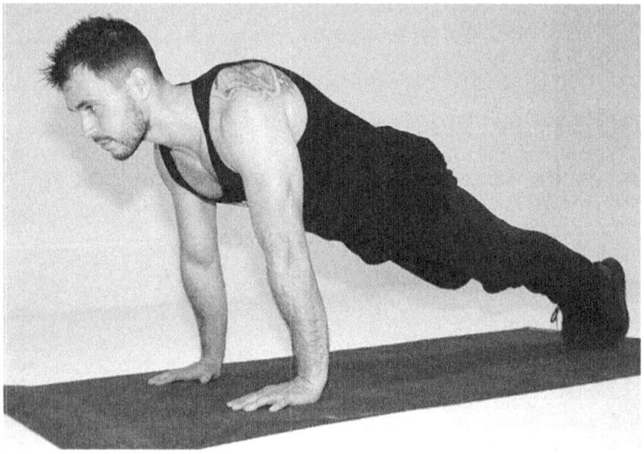

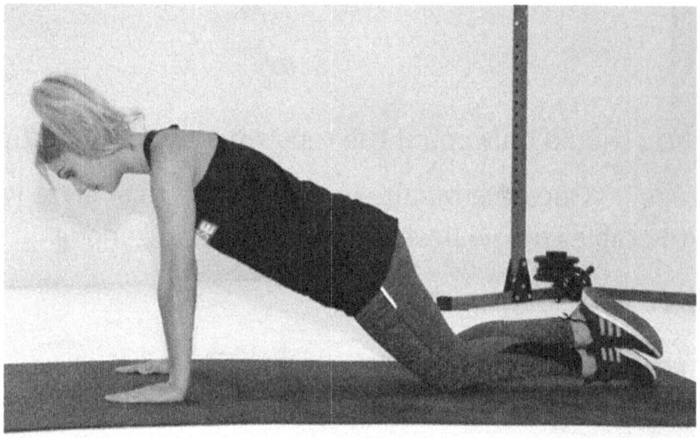

Once you know the proper form, perform as many reps as you can in one minute and record your result.

When your minute is up, take a look at the tables below to see how well you did based on your age and gender:

MEN - TRADITIONAL VERSION OF THE PUSH-UPS (ON TOES)

Rating	20-29	30-39	40-49	50-59	60+
Excellent	> 54	> 44	> 39	> 34	> 29
Good	45-54	35-44	30-39	25-34	20-29
Average	35-44	24-34	20-29	15-24	10-19
Poor	20-34	15-24	12-19	8-14	5-9
Very Poor	< 20	< 15	< 12	< 8	< 5

WOMEN- MODIFIED PUSH-UPS (ON KNEES)

Rating	20-29	30-39	40-49	50-59	60+
Excellent	>48	>39	>34	>29	>19
Good	34-48	25-39	20-34	15-29	5-19
Average	17-33	12-24	8-19	6-14	3-4
Poor	6-16	4-11	3-7	2-5	1-2
Very Poor	< 6	< 4	< 3	< 2	< 1

Figures based on Y's Way to Physical Fitness: The Complete Guide to Fitness Testing and Instruction (1989)

CARDIOVASCULAR FITNESS TESTS

3. THREE MINUTE STEP TEST

The only pieces of equipment you will need for this test are a stopwatch or a clock and a step. The height of the step should be about 12 inches. To perform this test, step up and down at a steady pace while alternating your feet. You should be keeping a four-beat cycle for the entire three minutes. Once the three minutes are up, rest for about five seconds and check your heart rate for 15 seconds. Then, multiply the number of beats by four to get your Beats Per Minute (BPM).

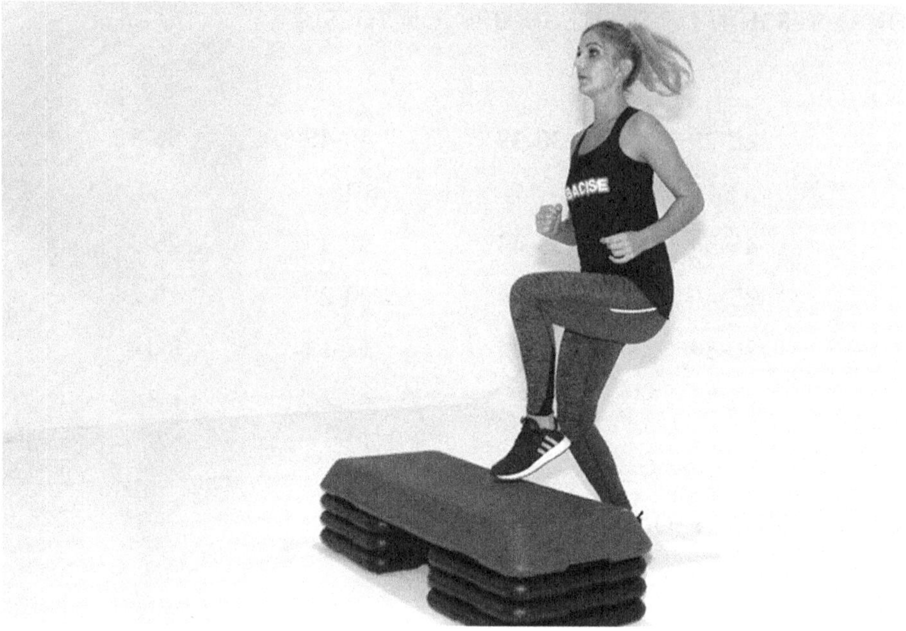

This test assesses your overall cardiovascular fitness and how quickly you recover. As we all know, the faster your heart rate returns to normal (also known as your resting heart rate), the better off you are. Once you find out your number of beats per minute, immediately after the three-minute step session, you will be able to examine where your result fits in.

To analyze your results based on your age and gender view the demographic averages via these tables:

MEN

Rating	**18-25**	**26-35**	**36-45**	**46-55**	**56-65**	**65+**
Excellent	50-76	51-76	49-76	56-82	60-77	59-81
Good	79-84	79-85	80-88	87-93	86-94	87-92
Above Average	88-93	88-94	92-88	95-101	97-100	94-102
Average	95-100	96-102	100-105	103-111	103-109	104-110
Below Average	102-107	104-110	108-113	113-119	111-117	114-118
Poor	111-119	114-121	116-124	121-126	119-128	121-126
Very Poor	124-157	126-161	130-163	131-159	131-154	130-151

WOMEN

Rating	18-25	26-35	36-45	46-55	56-65	65+
Excellent	52-81	58-80	51-84	63-91	60-92	70-92
Good	85-93	85-92	89-96	95-101	97-103	96-101
Above Average	96-102	95-101	100-104	104-110	106-111	104-111
Average	104-110	104-110	107-112	113-118	113-118	116-121
Below Average	113-120	113-119	115-120	120-124	119-127	123-126
Poor	122-131	122-129	124 132	126-132	129-135	128-133
Very Poor	135-169	134-171	137-169	137-171	141-174	135-155

Figures based on guidelines published by the American College of Sports Medicine (ACSM)

4. COOPER TEST

The Cooper test is a good way to measure your cardiovascular fitness. The purpose of this test is to see how far you can run in 12 minutes. If you're in the gym, you only need a treadmill to complete this test. You could also take this test by running outside. However, you would need an accurate way of measuring the distance you have covered as well as a stopwatch.

During the Cooper Test, you will want to try and run at a constant speed — or if you prefer, start off slow and end in a sprint! Be careful not to overexert yourself by running too fast at the beginning of the test.

A few words of caution: since this is a test of your cardiovascular fitness, it is best to get a physician's clearance prior to performing it. This test is not recommended for people with heart conditions, as there are risks associated with it. Additionally, you should also keep an eye on your heart rate to avoid extreme overexertion.

Use the following tables to see approximately where you stand based on your age and gender.

MEN

Age	Excellent	Above Average	Average	Below Average	Poor
Male 20-29	>2800m	2400-2800m	2200-2399m	1600-2199m	<1600m
Males 30-39	>2700m	2300-2700m	1900-2299m	1500-1999m	<1500m
Males 40-49	>2500m	2100-2500m	1700-2099m	1400-1699m	<1400m
Males 50+	>2400m	2000-2400m	1600-1999m	1300-1599m	<1300m

WOMEN

Age	Excellent	Above Average	Average	Below Average	Poor
Females 20-29	>2700m	2200-2700m	1800-2199m	1500-1799m	<1500m
Females 30-39	>2500m	2000-2500m	1700-1999m	1400-1699m	<1400m
Females 40-49	>2300m	1900-2300m	1500-1899m	1200-1499m	<1200m
Females 50+	>2200m	1700-2200m	1400-1699m	1100-1399m	<1100m

Figures based on Cooper Test by Kenneth H. Cooper (1968)

STRENGTH TESTS

5. SARGENT JUMP TEST

This test is designed to measure your leg strength and explosive power. It does this by measuring the distance (in centimeters) between your standing height and the height at which you can jump. All you need for this test is a wall, chalk and a tape measure. A ladder might come in handy, too, if you are not able to extend your tape measure upward far enough.

To perform this test, stand next to a wall sideways on. Extend your arm (closest to the wall) fully upwards and touch the wall with your fingertips. Either try to remember this spot or ask someone to assist you and chalk a line on the wall. This is your standing mark. Next, stand slightly away from the wall (so you don't scrape yourself) and then jump up as high as possible. Touch the wall at the highest part of your jump. Your result is the measurement between your standing mark and the highest point at which you touch the wall when jumping.

Don't forget to record your results in centimeters. You can take the highest measurement from three attempts for this test.

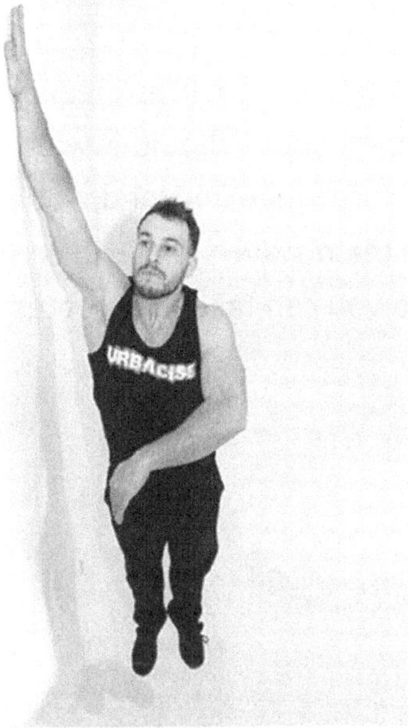

Rating	Men	Women
Excellent	>70	>60
Very Good	61-70	51-60
Above Average	51-60	41-50
Average	41-50	31-40
Below Average	31-40	21-30
Poor	8-12	11-20
Very Poor	<8	<11

Figures based on Y's Way to Physical Fitness: The Complete Guide to Fitness Testing and Instruction (1989)

The standing long jump test (also known as the broad jump test) is very similar to that of the Sargent Jump Test, as it also measures your explosive leg power. This time, instead of jumping high you need to jump long.

Using the same tape measure and chalk as the Sargent Jump Test, mark your starting position on the ground. Make sure your feet are about shoulder width apart, then, using a two-footed take off, jump forward as far as you can. Make sure when you land, you also land with both feet contacting the ground at the same time. Now measure the distance (again in centimeters) between your starting position and your end position. With this test, you can take the greatest distance after having three attempts.

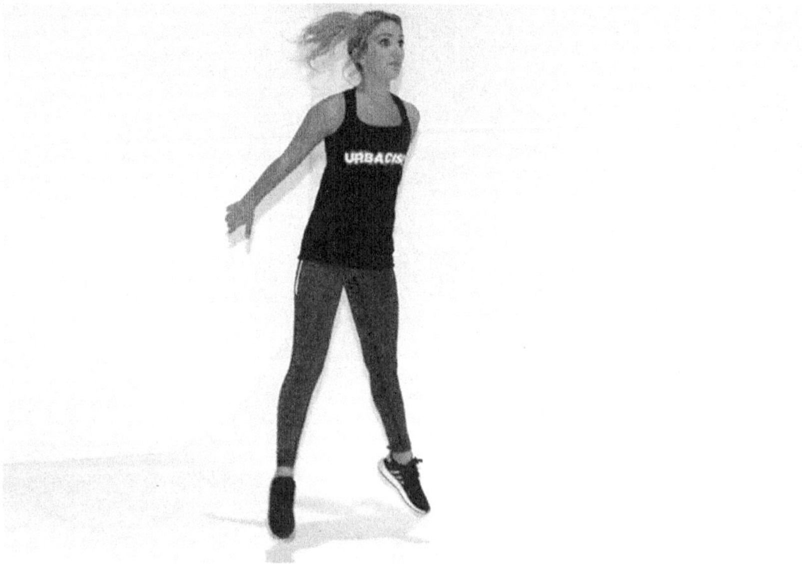

Rating	Men	Women
Excellent	>250	>200
Very Good	241-250	191-200
Above Average	231-240	181-190
Average	221-230	171-180
Below Average	211-220	161-170
Poor	191-210	141-160
Very Poor	<191	<141

Figures developed by Dr. Dudley Allen Sargent (1849-1924)

7. SIT AND REACH TEST

The sit and reach test is designed to measure the range of flexibility in your lower back and hamstrings. All you'll need for this test is a box (approximately 10 inches/30 cm high) and a tape measure. Please make sure you warm up before attempting this test as this test requires you to flex your back and hamstrings as much as possible. If you haven't warmed up beforehand, the chances of pulling a muscle are increased.

To perform this test, start by taking your shoes off and sitting on the floor. Sit with your legs straight/fully extended and your knees locked out, with the soles of your feet flat against the side of the box. Now in a slow movement reach forward as far as possible. Record your results in centimeters. The edge of the box that's closest to you would be the 0 cm mark.

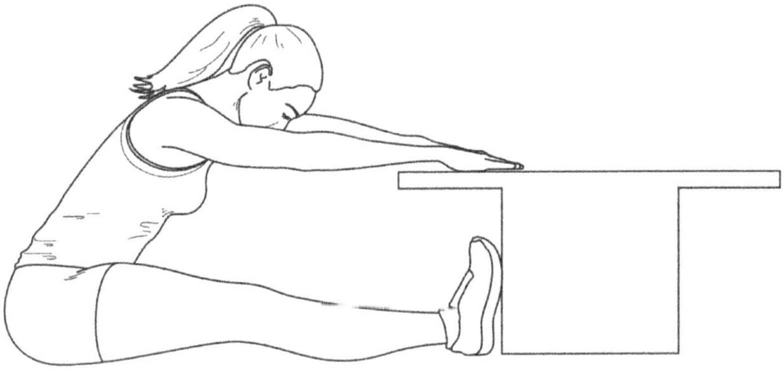

You need to hold the stretch for a count of three, so make sure you're not bouncing. You can take the greatest measurement from three attempts. Compare yourself to the average via this table:

Rating	Men	Women
Excellent	>17	>21
Good	+6 to +16	+11 to +20
Average	0 to +5	+1 to +10
Fair	-8 to -1	-7 to 0
Poor	-20 to -9	-15 to -8
Very Poor	< -20	< -15

Based on guidelines published by the American College of Sports Medicine (ACSM)

As you can see, the results of fitness tests always depend on your age and gender. For example, the number that's considered to be "excellent" for a 40-year-old woman would be considered "poor" for a 24-old-man. If you are conducting these fitness tests for the first time, please take your result with a pinch of salt. If you get a result that's considered "below average" for your age and gender, you can use it as an opportunity to improve. It is recommended that you try these fitness tests once every six weeks to track your progress and ensure that you are consistently working to improve your fitness.

CHAPTER TWO: STRUCTURING A WORKOUT PROGRAM

After determining your short, medium and long-term fitness goals and understanding your baseline fitness through testing, we can now move on to understanding and building an actual exercise program.

CHOOSING A SPLIT

When structuring an exercise program, the first thing you need to consider is how many days a week you're available to train. Then you can decide on different types of training days. You've no doubt heard the phrase "skipping leg day" — well, there are other days you shouldn't skip either.

"Leg day" is a classic component of a split workout. In essence, you're splitting your workout over different days and focusing on different parts of the body each day. There are a few variations of split workout programs, but we'll be looking at the main three:

- **Full-body split** - This is a good starting point if you're not an avid gym-goer and aim to work out three times a week or less. But please note: this split is not merely for beginners and can still be used for more advanced programs.
- **Upper/Lower split** - This program allows you to push the upper and lower body equally while making it easy to manage your workouts. This split is recommended for training four times a week.
- **Push/Pull/Leg split** - The most efficient split we'll be covering allows you to train opposing muscle groups separately for maximum overload. This is recommended if you want a more advanced program, training five times a week.

1. FULL-BODY SPLIT ROUTINE

If you're relatively new to exercise or want good overall fitness, a full-body training session could best-suit you. Full-body training is less targeted than the other two splits we'll be looking at, as it targets your whole body. This means it's harder to overload your muscles. It's also easier to burn yourself out using the full-body split if you don't take enough time to recover between workouts. For instance, if you work out two days in a row using this method, your muscles will most likely not be fully recovered. You'll soon start developing signs of overtraining, and your workouts won't be as effective. A full-body split can also take more time per session, so this split may not be the best if you have a busy schedule.

An example of a full-body split week would be:

Mon	Tue	Wed	Thurs	Fri	Sat	Sun
Full body	Rest	Full body	Rest	Full body	Rest	Rest

On a full-body split day, you would work all your muscle groups in the same session: quadriceps, glutes, hamstrings, calves, back, biceps, chest, shoulders and triceps.

Later, we'll provide some example exercises and tell you the optimal order to put these exercises in.

2. UPPER/LOWER SPLIT

The next split is the upper/lower split, where you work the upper and lower parts (legs & core) of your body on separate days.

This is not as efficient as the push/pull/leg split that we'll get to next. Here, you are combining rear and front muscle groups, making it harder to overload your muscles as effectively. However, this is good if you're looking to build muscle and if you're happy with a more general approach. This split allows your body to rest more than the full-body split. On the days you're working the upper portion of your body, your legs are recovering. And vice versa when you're working your legs.

An example of the upper/lower split week might look like this:

Mon	Tue	Wed	Thurs	Fri	Sat	Sun
Upper	Lower	Rest	Upper	Lower	Rest	Rest

On the lower split day, you would exercise your quadriceps, glutes, hamstrings, and calves.

MUSCLES WORKED ON LOWER SPLIT DAYS

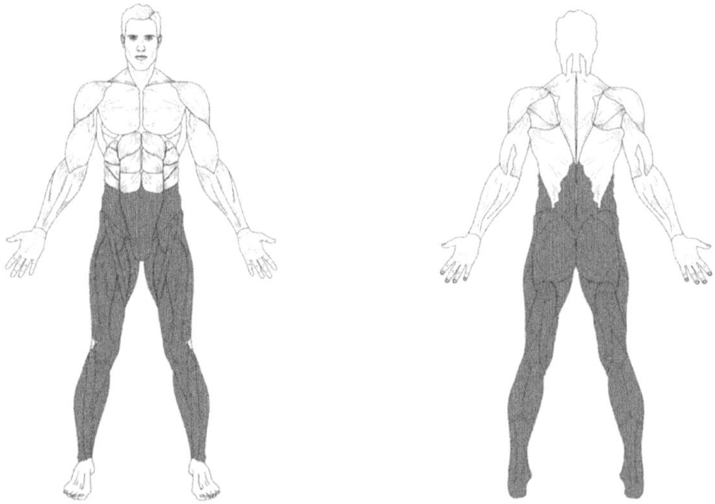

On the upper split day, you would exercise your back, biceps, chest, shoulders and triceps.

MUSCLES WORKED ON UPPER SPLIT DAYS

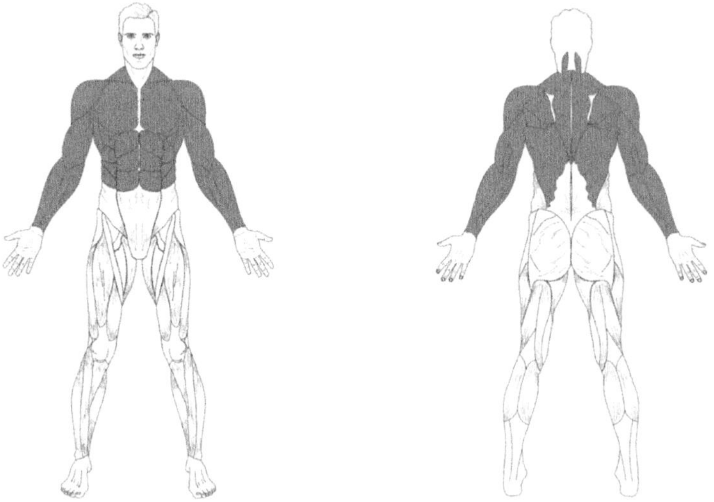

Example exercises to follow in a later chapter.

3. PUSH/PULL/LEG SPLIT

This split is designed to optimally train your muscles. It separates out your rear and front muscle groups so you can achieve greater overload.

- **Push day** - You concentrate on exercises where you need to push away from your body, working your chest, shoulders and triceps.

EXAMPLE OF A PUSH EXERCISE - PUSH-UP (PUSHING AGAINST THE GROUND)

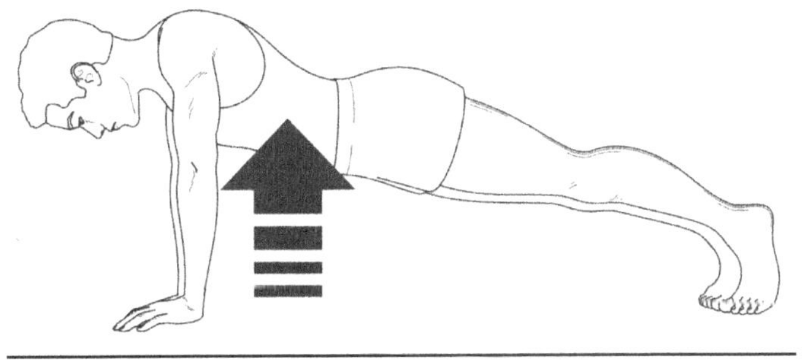

The push-up is a good example of a push exercise; another popular example would be the bench press.

EXAMPLE OF A PUSH EXERCISE - BENCH PRESS (PUSHING UPWARDS)

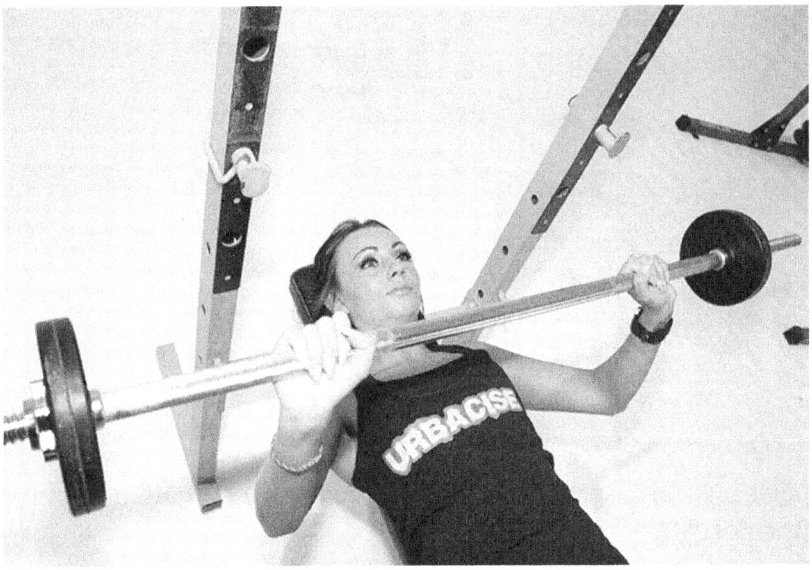

MUSCLES WORKED ON PUSH DAYS

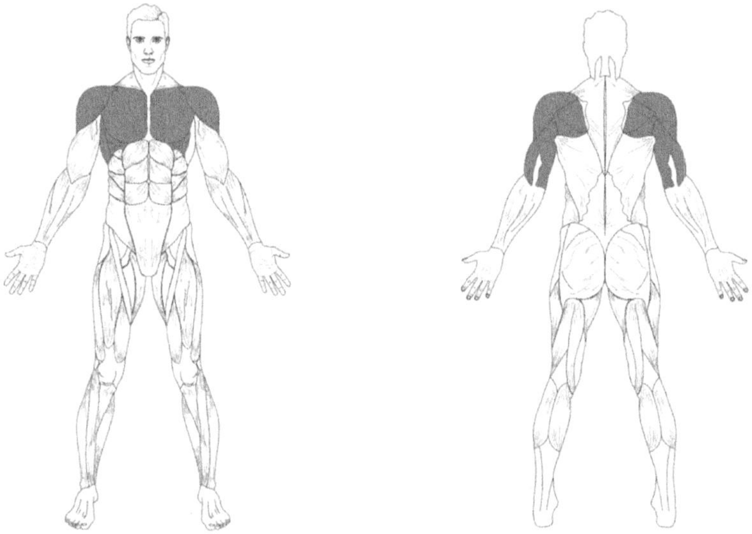

- **Pull day** - You focus on exercises that pull towards your body, working your back and biceps.

EXAMPLE OF A PULL EXERCISE - SEATED CABLE ROW (PULLING WHILE SEATED)

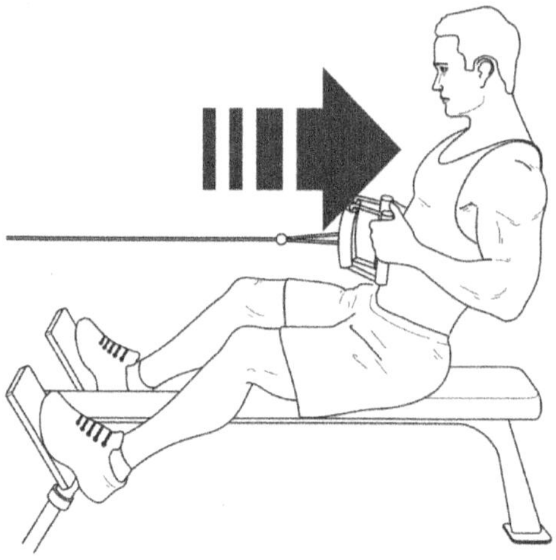

An example of a popular pull exercise would be the Seated Cable Row. Other examples include pull-ups, bent over rows and the deadlift.

EXAMPLE OF A PULL EXERCISE - DEADLIFT (PULLING WHILE STANDING)

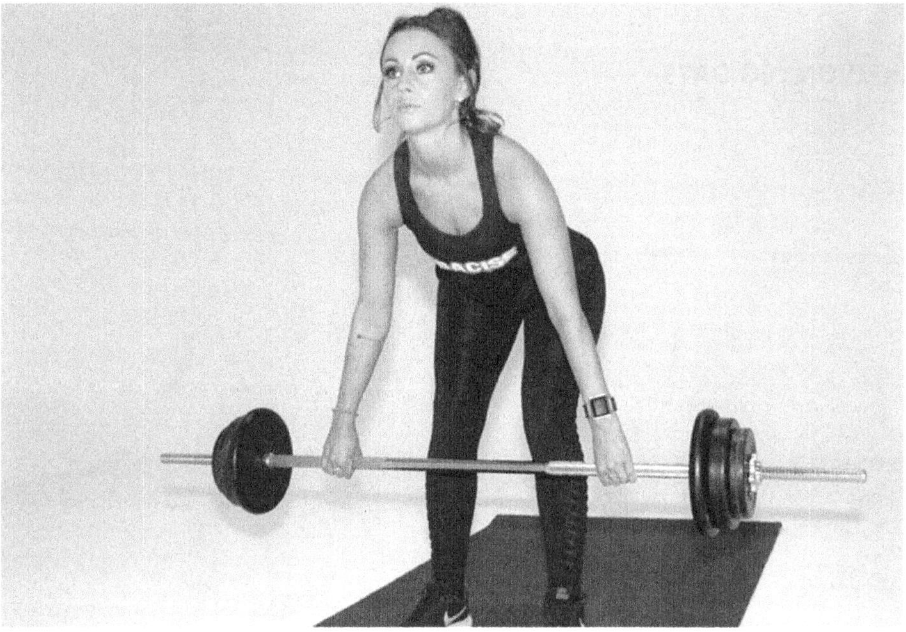

PLEASE NOTE: Deadlifts can also be performed on leg days, as it's a popular exercise for your hamstrings.

MUSCLES WORKED ON PULL DAYS

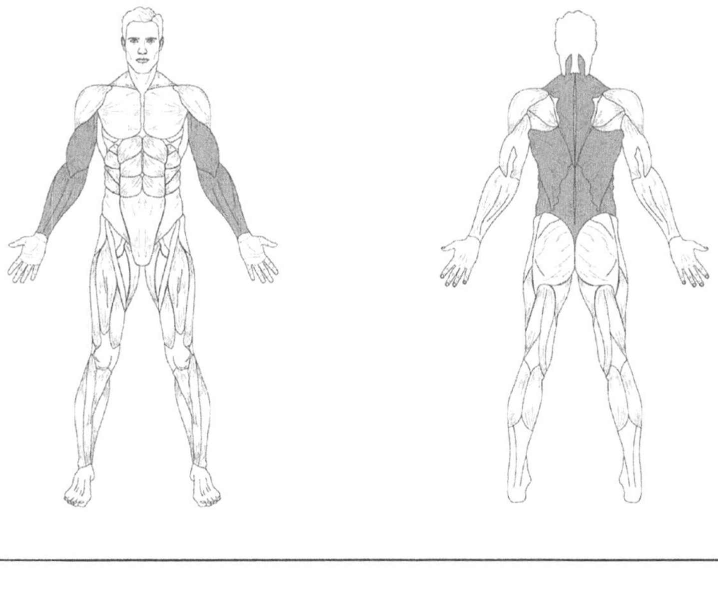

- **Leg day** - works your quads, glutes, hamstrings and calves.

MUSCLES WORKED ON LEG DAYS

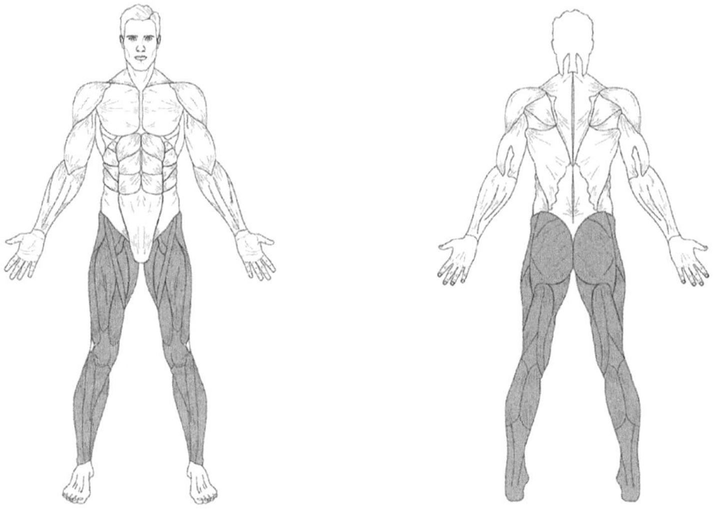

With this split, "Leg day" doesn't separate front and rear muscles. However, there is a logical order you could put your leg exercise in, which we'll examine a bit later.

WHY USE THE PUSH-PULL STRUCTURE?

The main advantage of using this split routine is avoiding overstressing your body. Push-pull training enables you to train more often compared to the full-body split. It's recommended that you take 48 hours rest after training a muscle group, so it has time to recover. With a split routine, you can train a different muscle group the day after — for example, doing the "push" split on Monday and "legs" on Tuesday.

Push-pull training also works each muscle to the best of its ability and achieves greater overload, as you are concentrating on that muscle as opposed to your full body. In a full-body workout, it would be quite hard to fully train each muscle in an optimal way as your body would become fatigued, causing your supporting muscles to be too tired to be worked at maximum effort.

If you choose to write your program based around the push/pull/leg split, your week might look a little bit like this:

Mon	Tue	Wed	Thurs	Fri	Sat	Sun
Pull	Legs	Push	Rest	Pull	Push	Rest

You can rotate the structure of this split each week. Why? It's recommended that you hit each muscle group twice a week. If we kept the above format, we would only be working the legs once that week. But if you rotate the days the next week, you might have an exercise program following this layout:

Mon	Tue	Wed	Thurs	Fri	Sat	Sun
Legs	Pull	Push	Rest	Legs	Pull	Push

You are now working your legs twice within the same seven-day period.

With this example, you can mix it up, switch the days around, and move your rest days in between your workout days so it fits your schedule and recovery.

PULL BEFORE YOU PUSH

It's always recommended that you do a pull exercise before a push exercise, and you should also do more pull exercises than push. The main reason for this is to prevent imbalances between your opposing muscle groups, which can result in injury. The muscles in the front of our bodies are normally stronger (e.g. biceps, quadriceps, chest), as we use them more in our daily activities. If a person's chest is more developed than their back (which is often the case), this can lead to back pain or injury.

Another important aspect of doing more pull exercises, in general, relates to your "scapular stability." The scapular, also known as the shoulder blade, is responsible for the movement of the shoulder. When doing push exercises such as a bench press, it's easy to injure your rotator cuff if your scapular muscles aren't strong and well-supporting.

DIAGRAM OF THE SCAPULAR

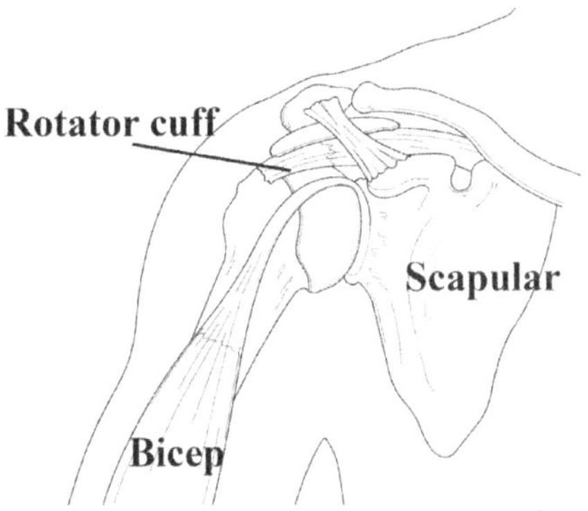

You might have noticed in all these splits that we have not spoken much about the core. Although in this book we'll just be referring to your core as one muscle group, the core actually includes your glutes, hips, abdominal muscles, inner abdominal muscles, pelvic floor and scapula.

In general, people tend to exercise their core on the "lower" or "leg" day. However, you can exercise it every day, if you wish. Alternatively, you might choose to have a separate day altogether for your core exercises, depending on your preference and goals.

When performing core or ab work, remember to do exercises that target both front and back muscles (like push/pull). An example of this would be doing sit-ups (***Figure 1)*** for your front followed by a superman (***Figure 2)***, which is a back exercise.

Figure 1: Sit-Up

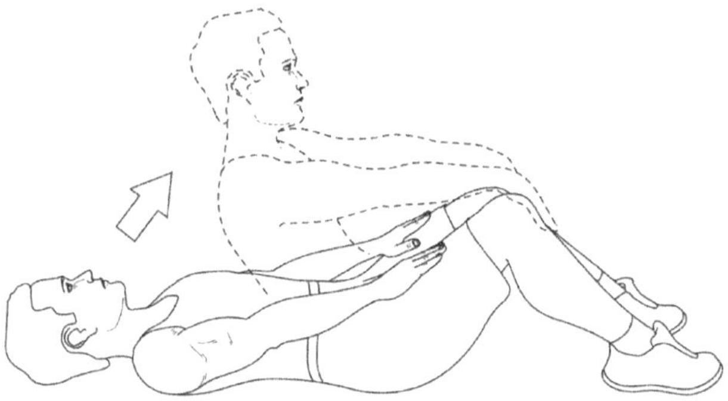

Figure 2: Superman

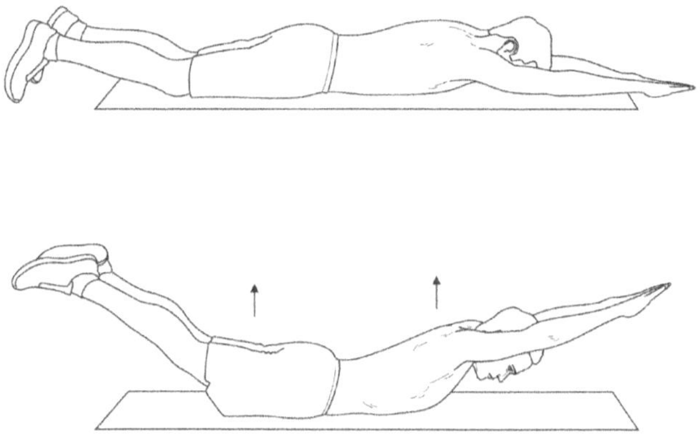

This diagram shows the muscles we are referring to when we mention the core:

MUSCLES WORKED FOR CORE

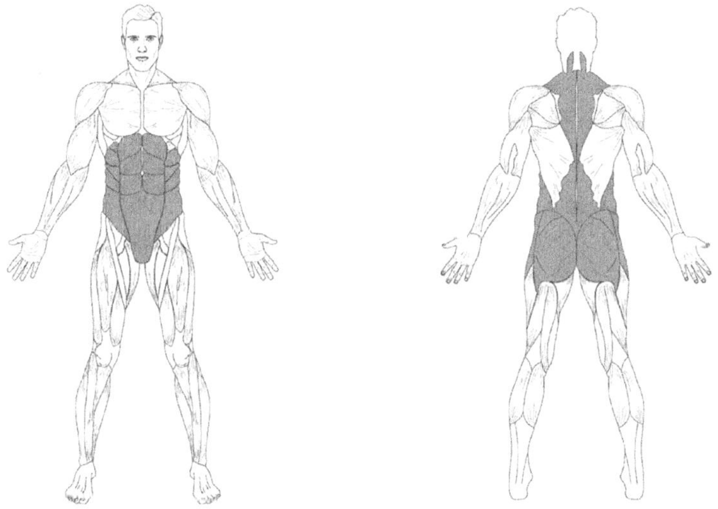

HIT MUSCLE GROUPS TWICE A WEEK

With any of these splits, it's up to you to decide how frequently you work out. However, as previously mentioned, it is recommended that you hit each muscle group at least twice a week. If you are only training a muscle group once each week, your progress in strength and fitness won't be as noticeable. On the flip side, hitting a muscle group three or more times a week can lead to overtraining or the neglecting of other muscle groups. For example, if you do upper body four times a week and legs only one day a week, this will lead to imbalances, or worse "chicken legs"! Hitting a muscle group twice a week is optimal and can be achieved using any of the splits.

THE SCIENCE BEHIND THE SPLIT WORKOUT

In order to understand the science behind these splits, particularly the push/pull/leg split, you need to know a little bit about biology and how the body works.

Muscles are designed to contract and relax. That's their main function. Muscles stretch over joints, which enables us to move our limbs. Responsible for moving each joint are two opposing muscles. Push and pull exercises hit these two opposing muscles, known as agonist and antagonistic pairs of muscles.

- **Agonist** - The muscle that moves while performing an exercise
- **Antagonistic** - The muscle that opposes the agonist muscle

The below image helps to demonstrate the agonist and antagonistic muscles in more detail. Take the arm as an example., your arm can move because of the opposing forces from your biceps and triceps.

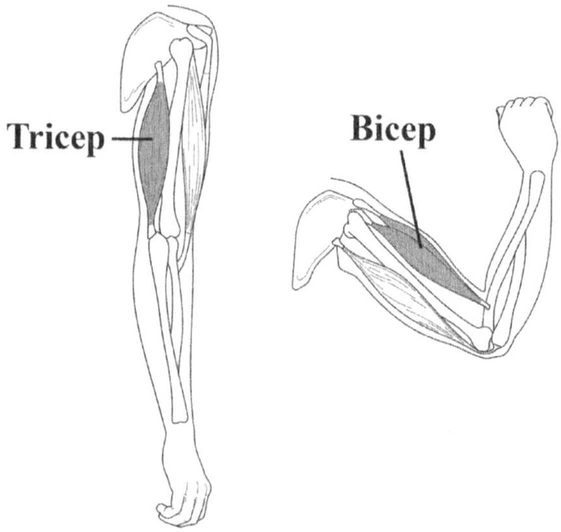

With a tricep dip exercise (***Figure 4***), your triceps would be the agonist muscle (the main muscle being developed) and your bicep the antagonistic. With a bicep curl exercise (***Figure 5***) the roles would switch.

Figure 4: Tricep Dip

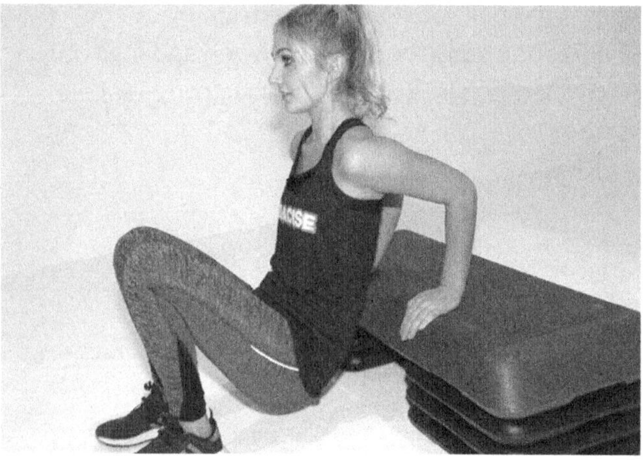

Figure 5: Bicep Curl

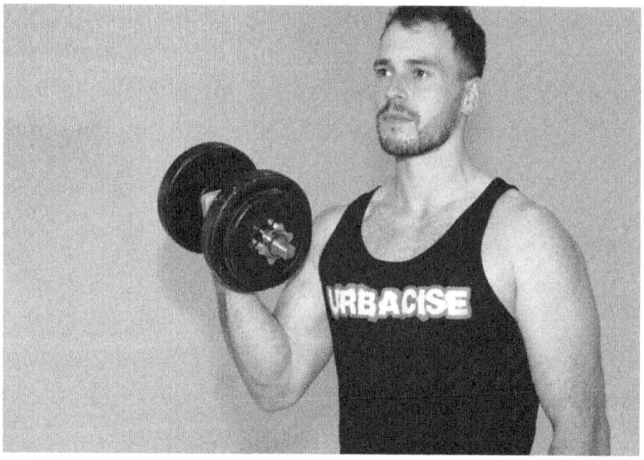

Here's a list of the agonist and antagonistic pairs in the human body. Please note: after this section, we'll be referring to these muscle groups by their muscle group name (i.e. "back") as opposed to their more scientific individual names. This is for the sake of simplicity.

Biceps (Arm)	**PAIRED WITH**	Triceps (Arm)
Deltoids (Shoulder)	**PAIRED WITH**	Latissimus Dorsi (Back)
Pectoralis Major (Chest)	**PAIRED WITH**	Trapezius/Rhomboids (Back)
Rectus Abdominis (Abs)	**PAIRED WITH**	Erector Spinae (Back)
Iliopsoas (Hip)	**PAIRED WITH**	Gluteus Maximus (Hip)
Quadriceps (Thigh)	**PAIRED WITH**	Hamstrings (Behind the knee)
Hip Adductor (Hip)	**PAIRED WITH**	Gluteus Medius (Hip)
Tibialis Anterior (leg)	**PAIRED WITH**	Gastrocnemius (leg)

We'll be talking about agonist and antagonistic pairs of muscles more when we discuss supersets — more advanced ways of exercising — a little bit later.

Further reading: the appendices contain the science behind the methods described within each section. This will mean you can skip the science parts and just use the main step-by-step guide of how to write an exercise program (if you desire).

CHAPTER THREE: DECIDE WHICH MUSCLES TO EXERCISE FIRST

Before we start looking at what exercises we need in our program, we need to determine what muscle group to exercise first. When looking at a "Push" day, for instance, do you put Skull Crushers (***Figure 6***) before or after Bench Press (***Figure 7***)? Or, in a full-body workout, would you exercise your legs at the start or the end of your session?

Figure 6: Skull Crusher

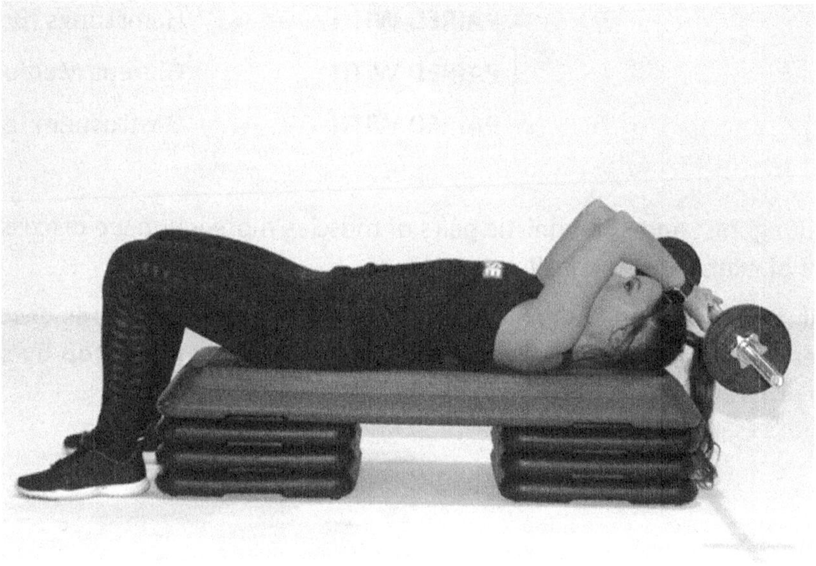

Figure 7: Bench Press

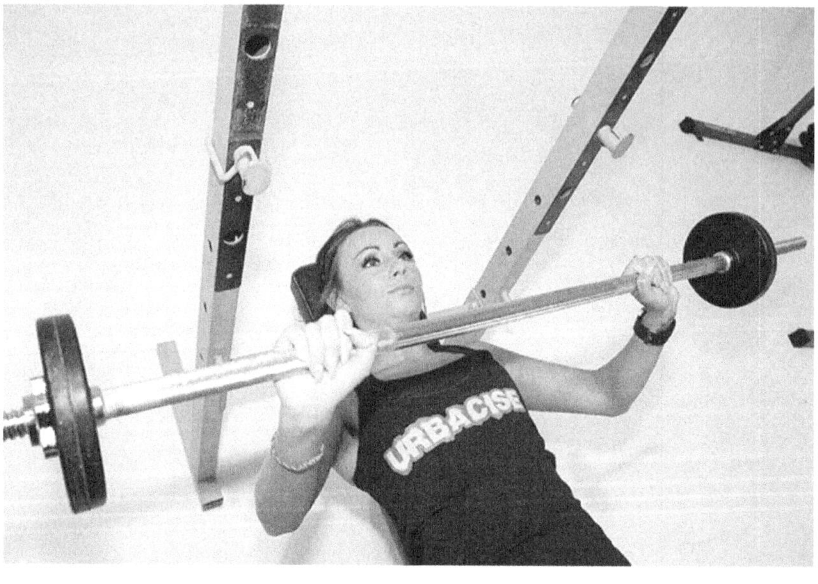

In anaerobic exercise (weight training), whether you're training for power, strength or size, the whole premise is to put your tendons under pressure, tiring them out and causing micro-tears to form so they repair themselves and grow back stronger and bigger. So, when thinking about the order to put your exercises in, you want to start with the exercise that tires out the biggest muscle first.

By exercising the biggest muscle first, you can overload it as much as possible while it's also being supported by the smaller muscles, also known as synergist muscles. This can aid in lifting heavier weight and gaining endurance, since you have more energy and therefore more power. In addition, injuries are more preventable since you are not as fatigued. After you have exhausted the biggest muscle, you can then go on to develop the synergist muscles.

If we were putting the size of the body's muscle groups in order, biggest to smallest, the list would look as follows:

1. Quadriceps
2. Glutes
3. Hamstrings
4. Back
5. Chest
6. Abs
7. Shoulders
8. Calves
9. Triceps
10. Biceps

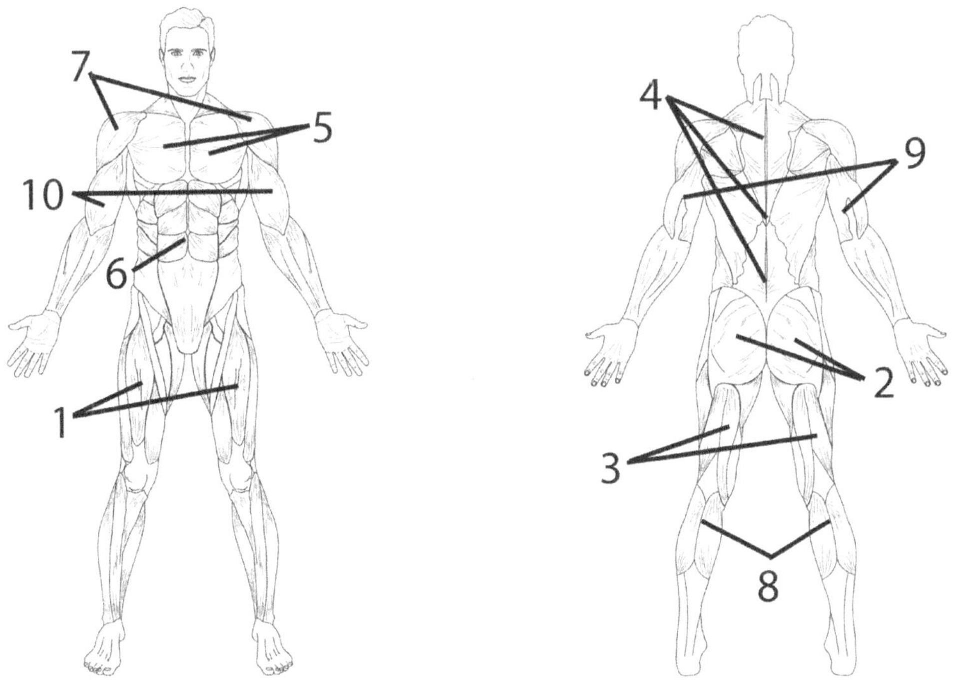

So, to answer our earlier question: **"Do you put Skull Crushers before or after Bench Press**?" You first need to know that a bench press exercises your chest and the Skull Crushers exercise your triceps. So, if we're exercising the biggest muscle first, you would put the bench press earlier in your workout than the skull crushers.

Here's an example of push exercises, if done in the below order we can see the muscle worked goes from largest to smallest:

1. 10 x Bench press **(chest)**
2. 10 x Push-ups **(chest)**
3. 10 x Military Press **(shoulders)**
4. 10 x Arnold Dumbbell Press **(shoulders)**
5. 10x Dips **(Triceps)**
6. 10 x cable pushdowns **(Triceps)**

You might be asking why I've put bench press in front of push-ups? Don't these two exercises work the same muscles? Bench press is for muscular strength, whereas push-ups are for muscular endurance. In general, bench press is a harder exercise (though this is dependent upon how much weight you put on the bar). A corollary to our basic rule for determining exercise order goes like this: start with the exercise that works the largest muscles and if there are two similar exercises, do the hardest one first. The reasoning behind this is simply:

- You have the most energy
- You are more focused

EXERCISE ORDER FOR A FULL-BODY SPLIT ROUTINE

With a full-body split, you would want to put the exercises in the order of the biggest muscles first. We know the biggest muscles of all are the quadriceps, so you'd want to put exercises that target those at the start of your program, such as:

- Leg Press
- Squats (***Figure 8)***
- Rope Jumping/Skipping (***Figure 9)***

Figure 8: Squats

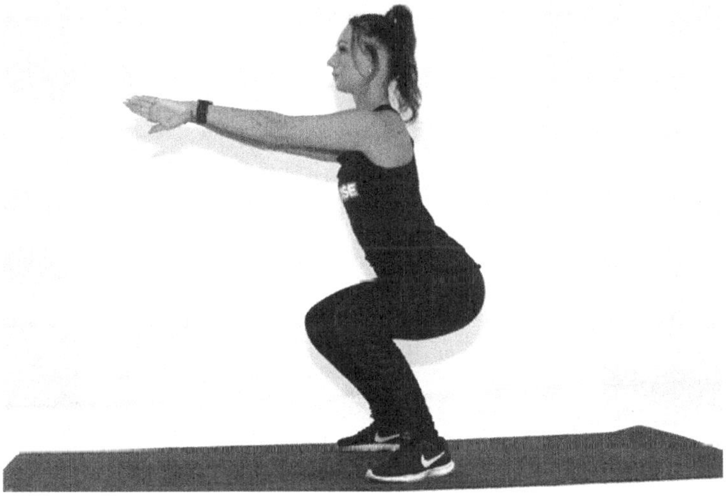

Figure 9: Rope Jumping/Skipping

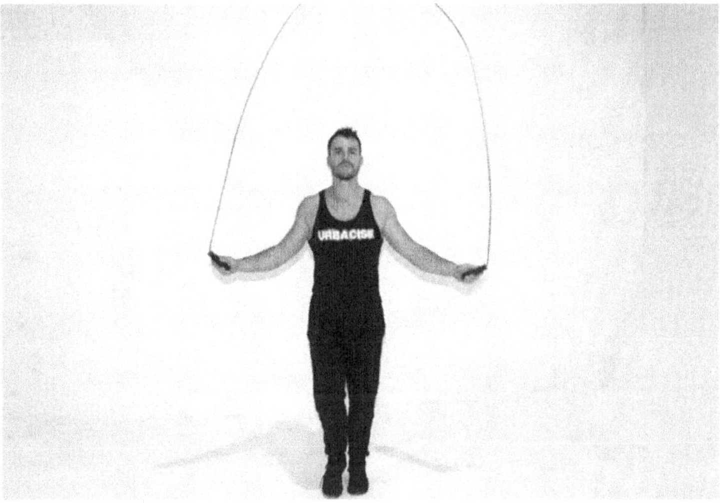

Then you could move onto the glutes and do exercises such as Barbell Hip Thrusts or Stiff-Legged Deadlifts. Then you just want to work your way down the list, finding exercises that target that muscle group: back, chest, abs, shoulders, etc.

Here's a simple workout that would exercise your whole body in a descending order of muscle group size:

- **Quadriceps** - Any type of squat, either bodyweight (***Figure 10)*** or weighted (***Figure 8).*** You can do jumping squats to make your workout harder.

Figure 10: Bodyweight Squat

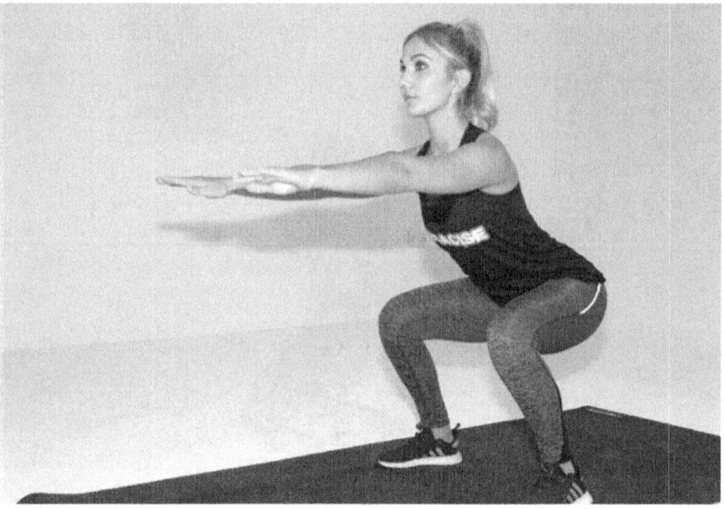

- **Glutes** - Bridging exercises (***Figure 11)*** whereby you lay on the floor with your legs bent and thrust upwards. You can also add weights to make this one harder.

Figure 11: *Glute Bridge*

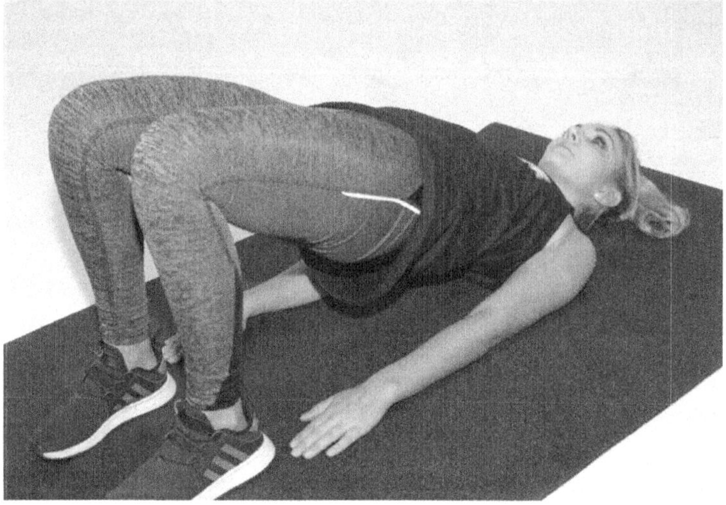

- **Hamstrings** - Stiff leg deadlifts (***Figure 12)*** with any kind of weight. If you can't perform exercises with weight for any reason, you could do a Walkout exercise or simply touch your toes.

Figure 12: Stiff Leg Deadlifts

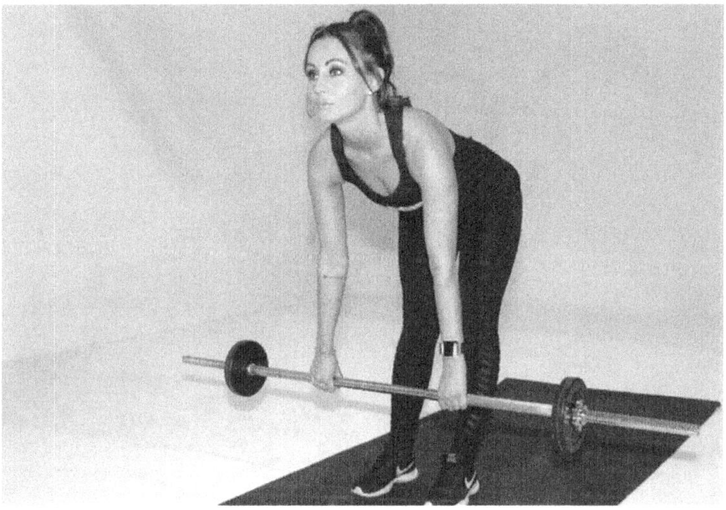

- **Back** - Bent over rows (***Figure 13)*** with weights, or if you're more athletic you could do pull-ups.

Figure 13: Bent Over Row

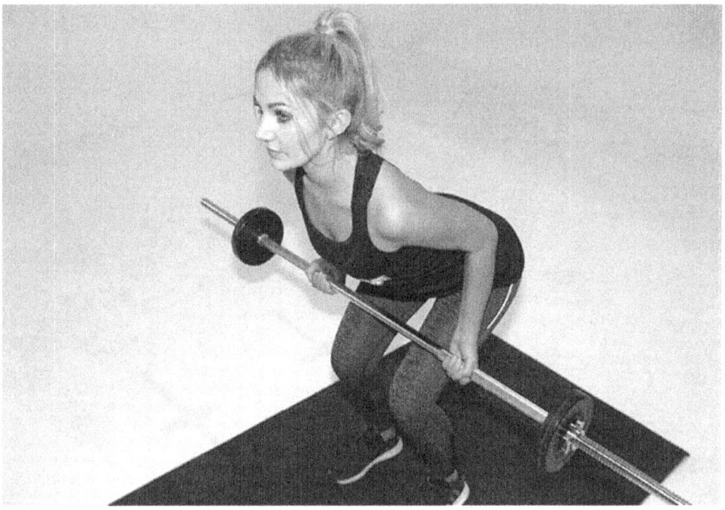

- **Chest** - Bench press is a popular one, but if you prefer an alternative that doesn't need any equipment, you could do push-ups (***Figure 14)*** or any push-up variation.

Figure 14: Push-Up

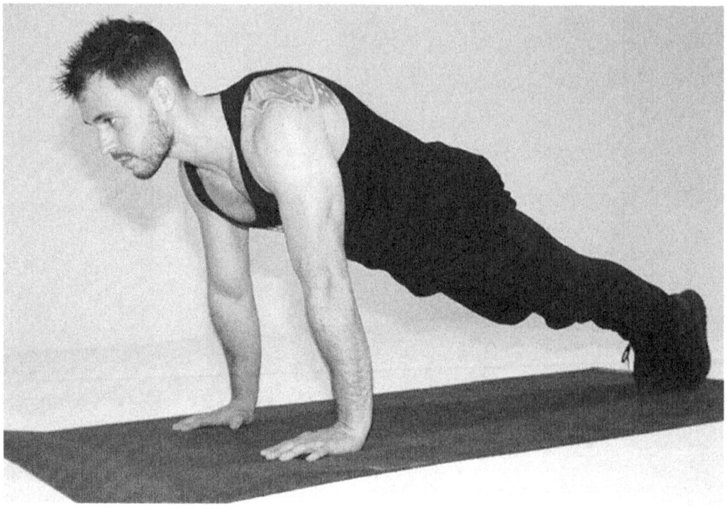

- **Abs** - There are so many ab exercises to choose from. The most popular are the plank (**Figure 15**), Russian twists, crunches, and leg lifts.

Figure 15: Plank

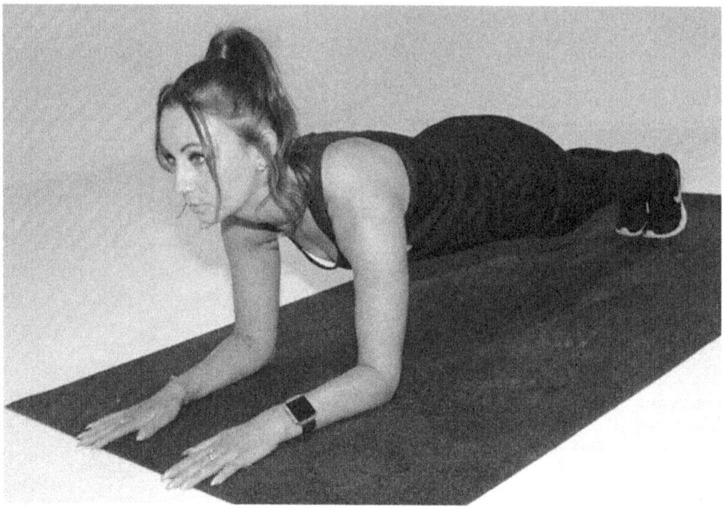

- **Shoulders** - Anything that involves lifting weight above your head. For example, power presses (**Figure 16**) with a barbell or dumbbells. If you're more athletic, you could do any kind of handstand variation (a wall handstand with shoulder taps, for example).

Figure 16: Barbell Power Press

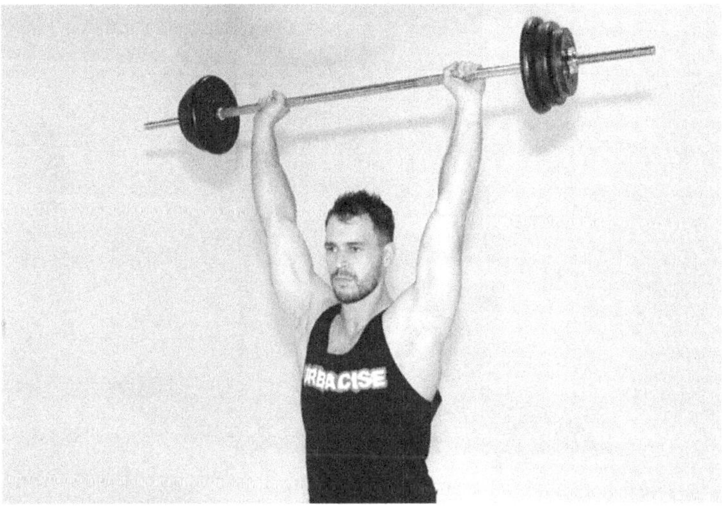

- Calves - The most popular one would be standing calf raises (**Figure 17**), adding weight to make it harder

Figure 17: Standing Calf Raises

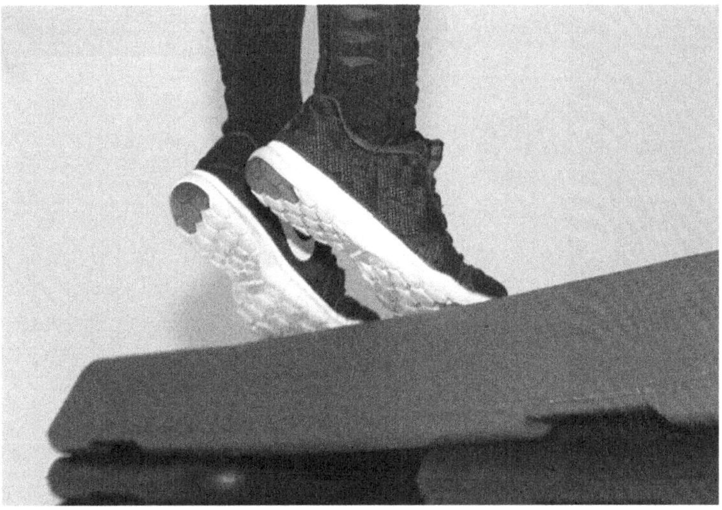

- **Triceps** - Any kind of dip, such as a bench dip.
- If you're not able to hold all of your bodyweight, you could do tricep extensions (**Figure 18**)

Figure 18: Tricep Extensions

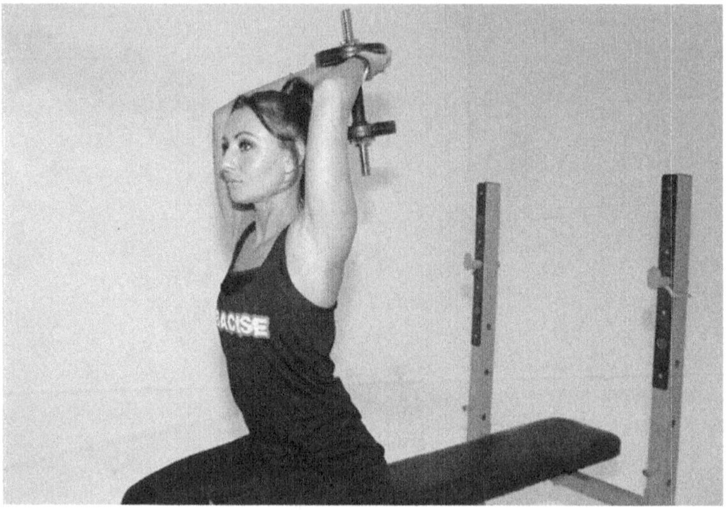

- **Biceps** - The most popular exercise is the bicep curl (**Figure 19**), either with dumbbells or a barbell.

Figure 19: Barbell Bicep Curl

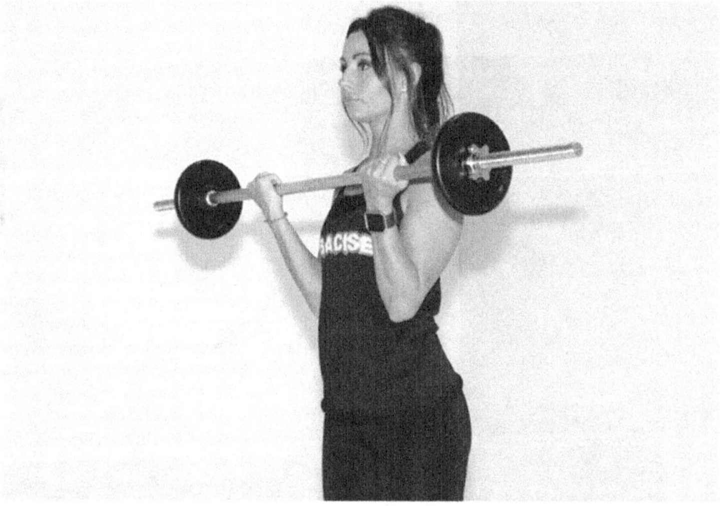

The above is a straightforward way of structuring and choosing exercises for a full-body workout. By the end of this book, you'll be able to incorporate more advanced techniques, such as a superset. You could use supersets to make your full-body workouts shorter in duration by training two muscle groups simultaneously (e.g., biceps and triceps). You can also rearrange certain muscle groups, for instance, you could move calves to the beginning of your workout by adding them to your warm-up. The reasoning for this would be that other exercises also train your calves, so it's not always necessary to work them individually. Another well-established structure of a full-body workout is moving your ab exercises to the end of the workout. This is because a lot of the other exercises also train your abs, so unless abs are your primary focus, you can train these last. Moving abs to the end of your workout also allows you to push yourself harder when working your shoulders, triceps and biceps.

COMPOUND EXERCISES & ISOLATION EXERCISES

Starting with the exercise that works the biggest muscle first is a good rule to follow, however there are subsets of that rule too. If you've heard a professional speaking about exercises, you might have heard the term "compound exercise" and wondered what these are. The opposite of a compound exercise is a "isolation exercise." It's easy to be confused by this terminology at first, however the difference between these two types of exercise is quite simple:

COMPOUND EXERCISES

Compound Exercises = Exercises that involve two or more different joints

Some common examples of compound exercises are:

- **Squats**
- **Deadlift**
- **Bench Press**

BARBELL SQUAT

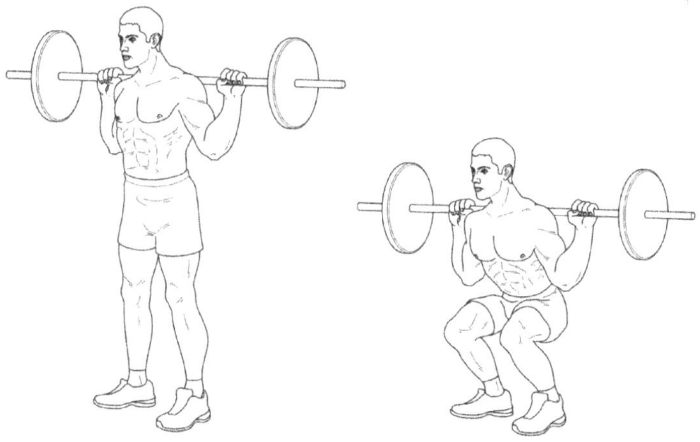

ISOLATION EXERCISES

Isolation exercises = Exercises that involve only one joint

Some common examples of isolation exercises are:

- Curls **(such a bicep curls)**
- Raises (**such a calf raises)**
- Flys **(such as the cable fly)**
- Extensions **(such as back extensions)**

BACK EXTENSION

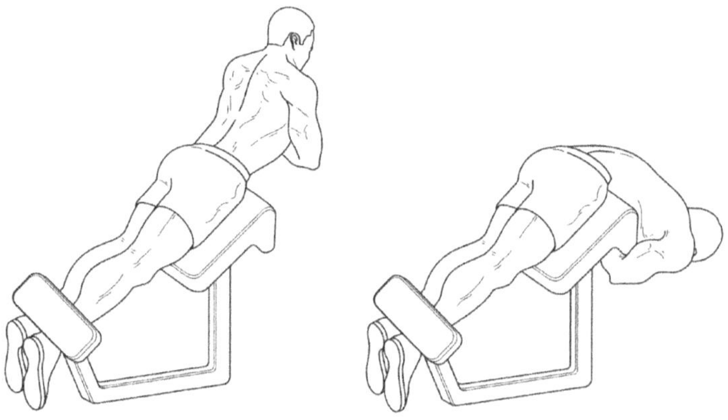

A lot of the machines you see in the gym tend to be isolation exercises.

When putting these two types of exercises into your program, you want to make sure that you put compound exercises in front of isolation exercises. A good example of this would be leg extensions and squats. We already know these exercises should come early on in your workout program, as they both work your quadriceps. However, based on the compound/isolation exercise information, we now know that squats come before leg extensions.

TARGETING A SPECIFIC MUSCLE

You might be asking, "What are the benefits of both compound and isolation exercises?" Compound exercises are great for targeting more than one muscle group, which helps to prevent imbalances. You could easily write an acceptable exercise program using compound exercises only. However, remember that the idea of working out (especially in a full-body split) is to tire your entire body; isolation exercises help you exhaust an individual muscle more, such as the smaller supporting muscles after you have worked the larger ones (for example, training your triceps after chest or biceps after back).

Some people want to exercise in order to obtain a certain look, for example: some ladies want their glutes to be proportionally bigger, and some guys want the same for their chest and biceps. This could be achieved by isolation exercises performed in a way that would cause hypertrophy (an increase in the size of muscle cells). You'd want to work your targeted muscle more than you do the other muscles.

For anyone who wants bigger glutes some of the best isolation exercises are:

- Glute Kickbacks

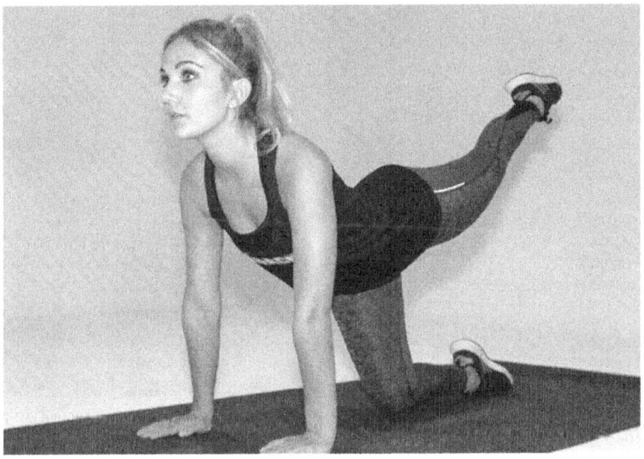

- Fire Hydrant

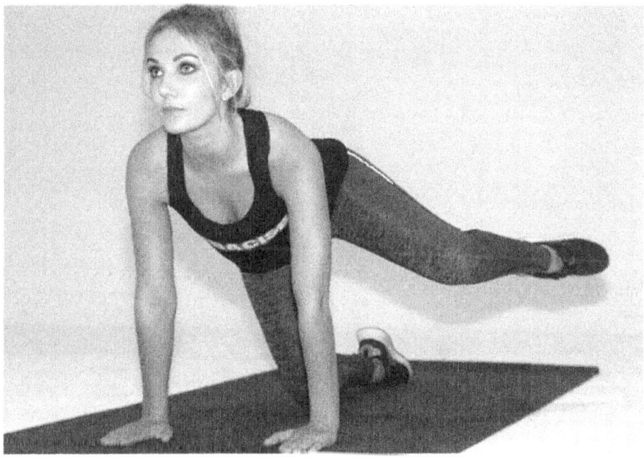

- Donkey Kicks

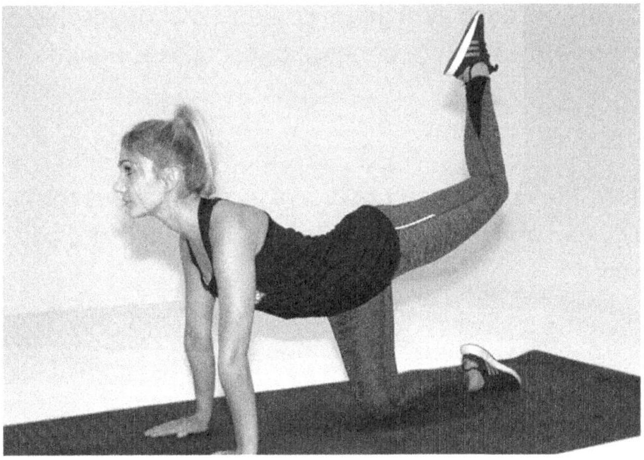

- Glute Bridges

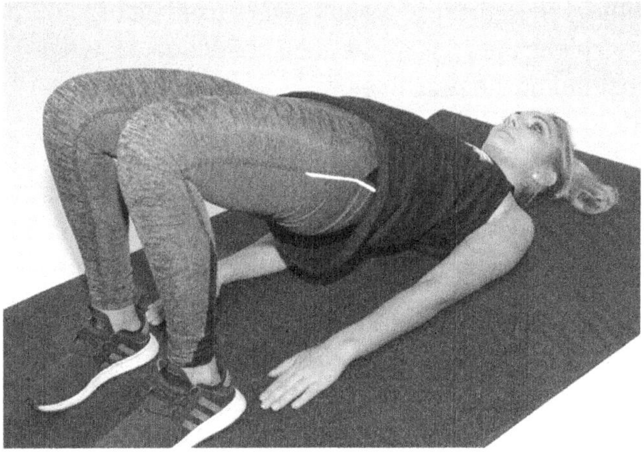

If you want a proportionally bigger chest and biceps, you could do:

- Cable Flys
- Chest Flys (***Figure 20***)
- Bicep Curl (***Figure 21***)

Figure 20: Standing Dumbbell Chest Fly

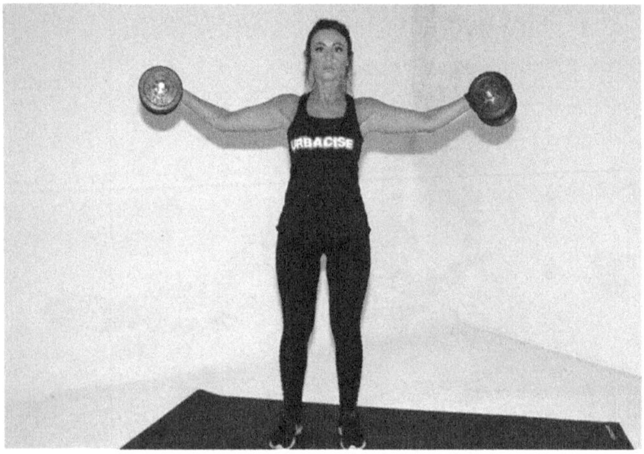

Figure 21: Bicep Curl

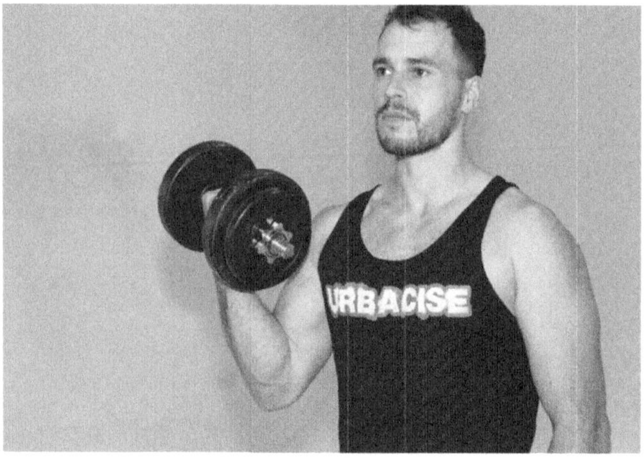

MACHINES OR FREE WEIGHTS FIRST?

When visiting a gym, you've probably seen someone lifting free weights in front of a mirror. For a long time, I thought free weights were used instead of machines because gym-goers couldn't maneuver the machines in order to see their reflection. However, it turns out there are benefits to using free weights instead of the machines.

- Exercise machines are good for beginners because they don't need to worry as much about form, reducing the risk of injury. If you're doing heavy clean and press exercises with a barbell, and you have bad form, it would be easy to hurt your back.
- Machines tend to focus on isolation exercises (like the leg press, for example), so you're only developing one muscle at a time.
- Machines can be good if you've developed imbalances in your muscles. Say, for example, your triceps are much stronger than your biceps. You can use the bicep curl machine to target just your bicep without it affecting your tricep as much as free weights would.

Free weights, however, allow you a greater range of motion (ROM), and your movements are more natural and in keeping with your normal daily activities. Free weights are also more effective for strength development as they also work the stabilizer muscles as opposed to individual muscles.

When writing your exercise program, make sure you work the biggest muscle first, then check if it is a compound or isolation exercise. If it's a compound exercise, put that exercise first, before isolation exercises. And put free weights before machine exercises.

For example, say you're targeting your back on a "pull day" and you're wanting to use the lat pulldown machine, but you also want to incorporate pull-ups into your session. Both are compound exercises, however pull-ups are harder, and you also aren't using a machine, so you'd put pull-ups before lat pulldowns.

For more information please see appendices:

Free Weights or Machines (Page 108)

CHAPTER FOUR: THE SIX FOUNDATIONAL MOVEMENT PATTERNS

We will now talk briefly about biomechanics. This is not to be confused with form. By now, hopefully you understand how important form is while exercising. If you do not know the correct form for an exercise visit our website for demonstration videos. (www.urbacise.com/exercises)

There are thousands of different exercises out there, many of which have confusing names or seem quite peculiar. It surprised me to learn that there are only six "foundational movement patterns." These are the universal ways that all humans move. These six foundational movements are:

1. Squat
2. Hinge
3. Lunge
4. Push
5. Pull
6. Carry

Learning these movements will help you to understand your body, make learning form easier and give you an understanding as to what's required in pre-workout stretching.

1. Squat. Many day-to-day activities require us to squat in one way or another. For example, in order to protect our backs, we need to squat down to pick up a heavy parcel off the floor. If you take an inventory of everything that you've done today, there is a good chance that you have needed to squat at some point.

Incorporating the squat into your exercise program should be relatively easy, because there are many variations of this movement. It's very important to pick the right variation of the squat, based on your ability to perform the move with proper form, to reduce your risk of injuries. Some variations of the squat include the bodyweight squat, jump squat, pistol squat, and barbell front and/or back squat. If you are new to squatting, you should start with the bodyweight squat and work your way up to more advanced variations of the move.

Figure 24: Barbell Squat

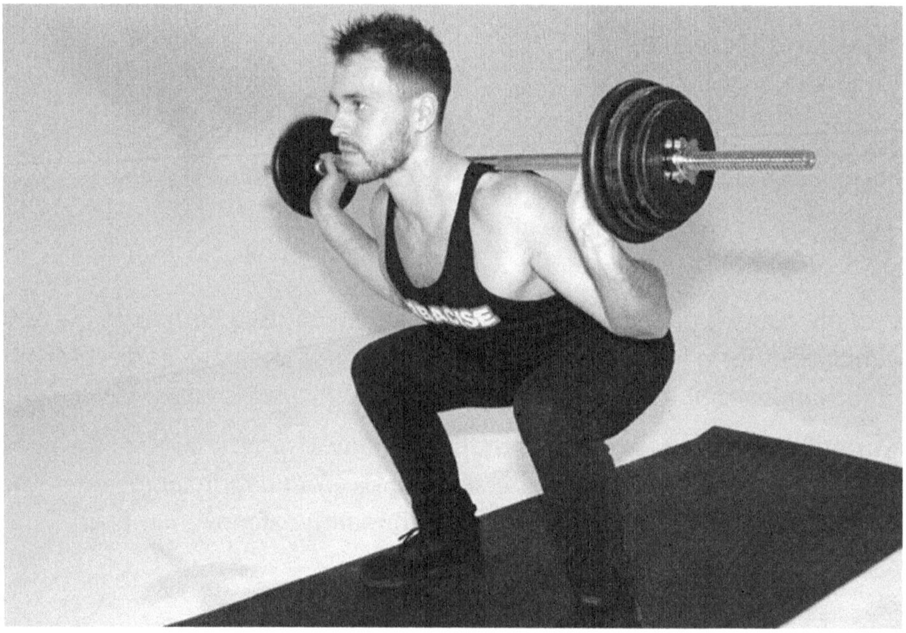

2. Hinge. To decrease the likelihood of lower back injuries from bending over throughout the day, it's very important that you master the hinge. Although the most famous hip hinge exercise is the barbell deadlift, it is not the only way to incorporate this movement pattern into your training. If this movement is not something you've practiced before, the barbell deadlift is not the best exercise for you, since you may be putting yourself at risk of an injury. Therefore, the first thing you should do to practice the hinge is to bend over without any weight (***Figure 25***). Once you are comfortable with bending over, try some light dumbbell deadlifts. Once the dumbbell deadlifts are easy, you can add the barbell deadlifts (***Figure 26***). Remember that proper form, above all else, is crucial when practicing the hip hinge.

Figure 25: Bend over with no weight

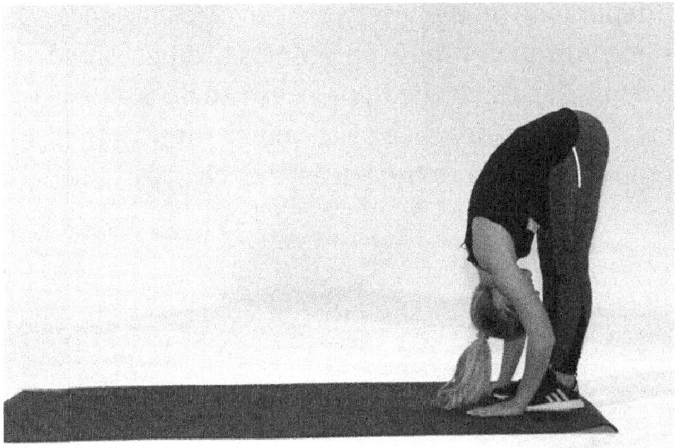

Figure 26: Barbell Deadlift

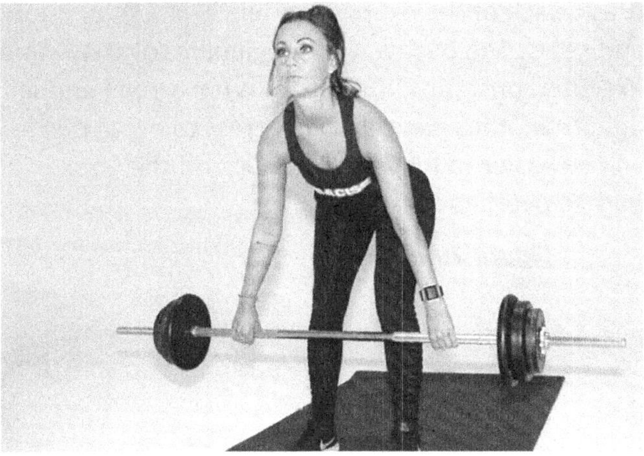

3. Lunge. The lunge (***Figure 28***) refers to a unilateral way of moving the lower body. Single-leg movement training is very important for day-to-day function. A lot of people, unfortunately, neglect single-leg movements. The reason why people don't often focus on any kind of unilateral training is that lunges are challenging and will amplify any muscle imbalances they may have.

People who do not have a lot of experience with lunges automatically think that they should be doing walking dumbbell lunges, which is not the case. In order to prevent potential knee, hip, lower back and ankle injuries, it's important to start with static single-leg movements before progressing to walking lunges. You can start with a combination of step ups (***Figure 27***) and bodyweight lunges to master the move. After that, you can progress to static weighted lunges and then walking lunges. It's important to make sure that you do the same number of repetitions on each leg in order to strengthen both legs equally.

Figure 27: Step Up

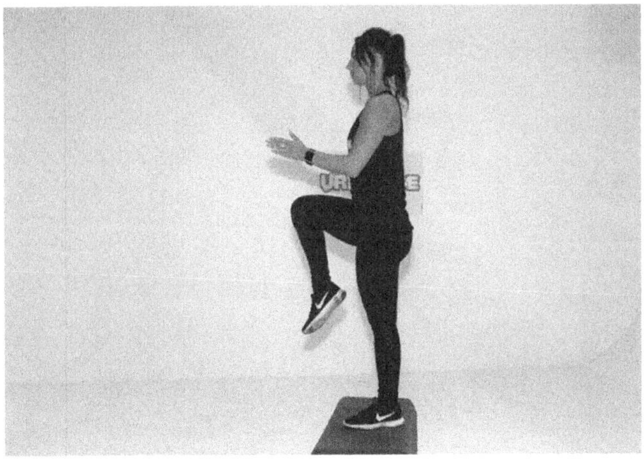

Figure 28: Lunge

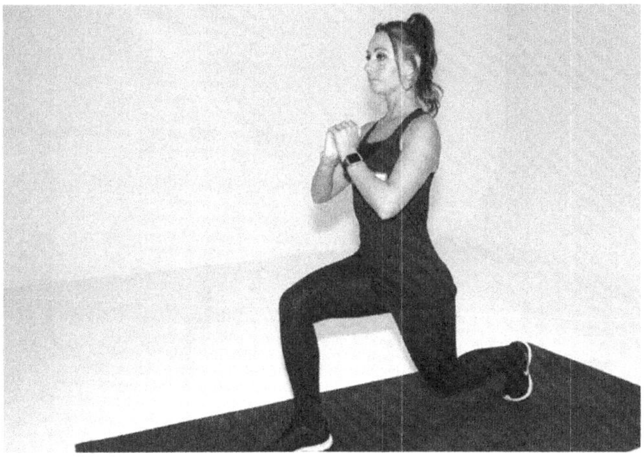

4. Push. The push (same as in the push/pull split) is an upper body movement that typically originates at the shoulder. The most common push exercises are the push-up (***Figure 29***), bench press and overhead press. Each of the exercises offers a variety of options, depending on the lifter's skill level, experience, and goals. The best way for beginners to integrate pushing into their fitness program is through properly executed push-ups. If a person is not strong enough to do push-ups off the floor, they can do wall push-ups. Then, they can slowly progress to doing push-ups with their hands on a solid bench. After that, it will be easier to move to push-ups off the floor — and then you're on to the barbell bench press and barbell overhead press.

Figure 29: Push-Up

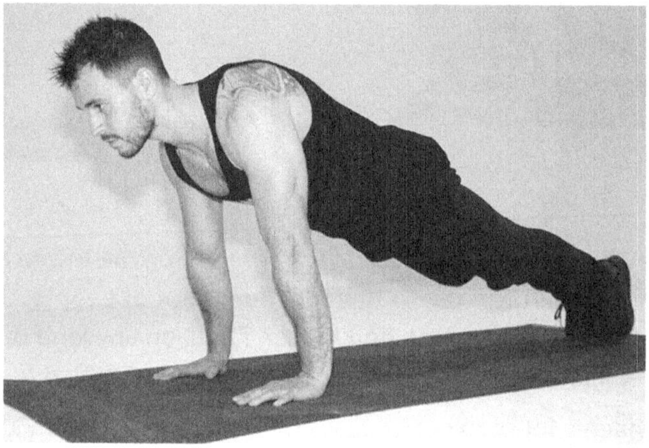

5. Pull. The pull (same as in the push/pull split) is another upper body movement that is critical for creating a strong and balanced back and biceps. One of the biggest mistakes that new lifters make is overdoing it on the push while neglecting the pull. This is common among guys who work on their chest more than their back. Whenever you think of the pull, you are probably thinking of the pull-up (***Figure 30***). However, the pull-up is a very advanced exercise and not everyone is strong enough to execute this move properly, though it is something to work towards. Knowing that the pull movement can be both vertical and horizontal, there are several exercises that will enable you to master this move. Some examples of pulling exercises include: inverted rows, dumbbell rows, bent over barbell rows, lat pull-downs and seated rows.

Figure 30: Pull-Up

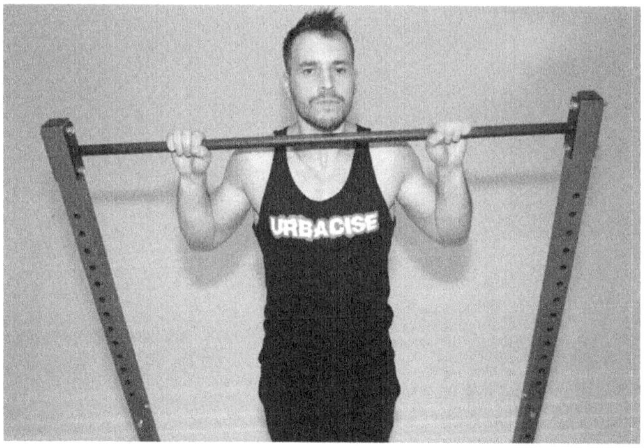

6. Carry. Contrary to popular belief, the carry is not all about carrying heavy loads while walking. Although the farmer's carry, hiking with a heavy backpack and carrying jugs of water in each hand are all examples of the carry, they are not the only options for practicing this move. In fact, the carry can be defined as moving your body forward, side-to-side and/or backward. It is not advised that you do any loaded carries if you have any dysfunctions in your body. First, you need to strengthen your core and learn how to walk properly. Once you've mastered walking and substantially increased your core strength, then you can walk while carrying a load. Other carry exercises that you can eventually incorporate into your routine include overhead carry (***Figure 31***), unilateral farmer's carry, front-loaded carry and farmer's carry.

Figure 31: Kettlebell Overhead Carry

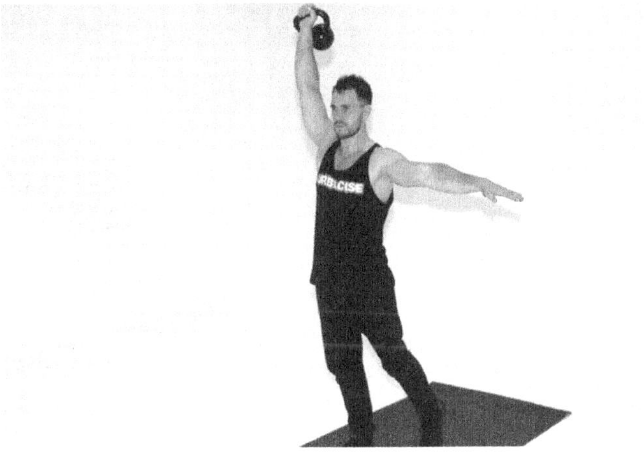

In order to get the best results, these are the six movements you'll be using throughout your exercise program.

Next, we'll be looking at stretching and how these foundational movement patterns help determine the type of stretching you should be doing.

REMEMBER TO STRETCH

Warming up and stretching is vital for preparing your body for physical activity. This is especially true if you sit at a desk all day or exercise right after waking up. Warm-ups prime your body for performance, preparing your brain and heart for exercise. Stretching is just as important in order to prevent soreness, decrease the risk of injuries and enhance performance.

It's recommended that you stretch both before and after your workout, so it's important to add stretches to your workout program. There are two types of stretches:

- **Dynamic** - These are stretches that mimic your actual workout and are based on the six foundational movement patterns. These include bodyweight lunges, squats and high knees.
- **Static** - These movements involve holding the stretch for a certain amount of time. Touching your toes for 30 seconds is an example.

It's recommended that you do dynamic stretches before your workout and static stretches in the cool down phase of your workout. As a develop your program, it might look a little bit like this:

Five minutes of dynamic stretching
Main workout program
Five minutes of static stretching

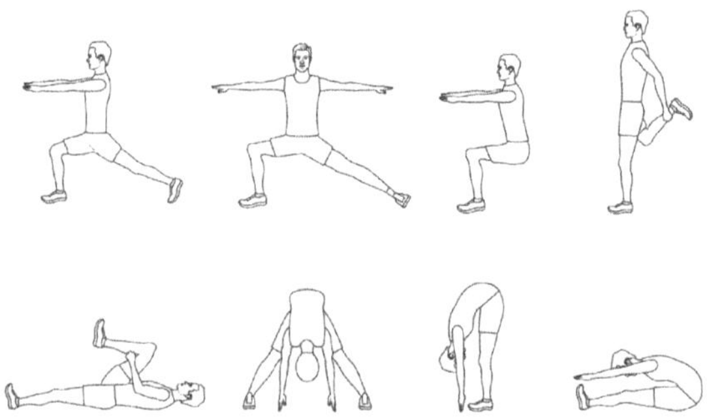

Example stretchers can be found on the website: www.urbacise.com/exercises

For more information please see appendices: Should I stretch before or after my workout? (Page 111)

CHAPTER FIVE: CHOOSE SOME EXERCISES

To help you better-understand the sort of exercise you should do for different muscle groups, let's get into a few examples. These examples are mixed in terms of their skill level to try and cater for all fitness levels. There are many more exercises that aren't on this list, you can find these on the Urbacise website: (www.urbacise.com/exercises).

We suggest you research different exercises and their variations - incorporating them into your workout.

IMPORTANT: once more it's important to state that if you are new to fitness training and you're not familiar with any of these exercises, you must make sure that you have the correct form. Otherwise, you are more susceptible to injury. So please, before you attempt to lift any heavy weights, make sure you know how to lift correctly.

Also, please make sure you are medically fit for any exercise training. I would suggest that if you're uncertain about your fitness level or you're having any trouble with any of the exercises, you get yourself a full medical examination.

Remember: the fitness tests at the start of this book can help you determine your baseline fitness. However, if you're in any doubt as to your abilities, I strongly suggest you see a medical professional.

QUADRICEPS EXERCISES

BODYWEIGHT LUNGE

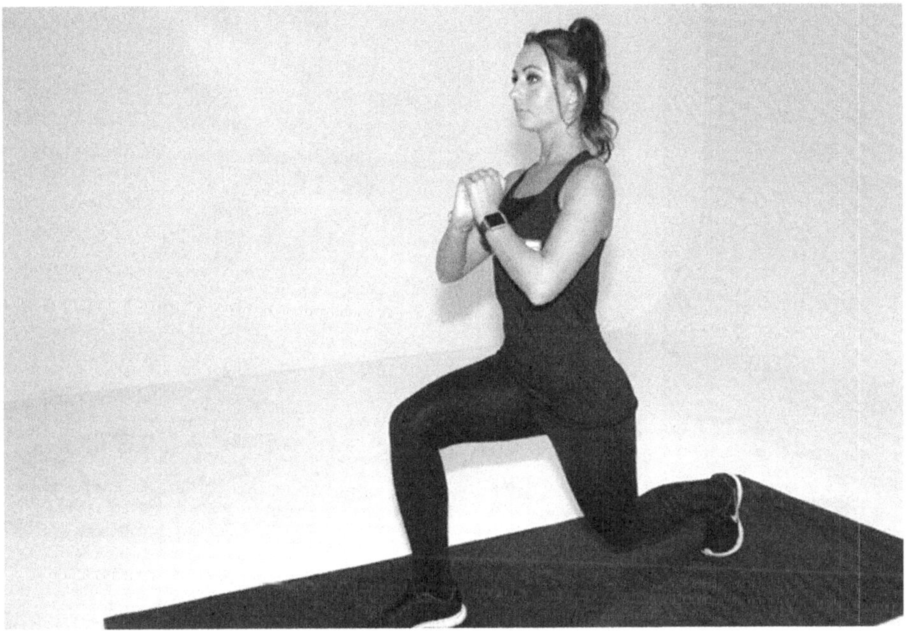

The lunge is a compound exercise that strengthens your quadriceps, glutes, hamstrings, and calves.

Lunges increase stability, balance, and flexibility of the body, which is helpful both in sports and everyday life. They effectively make your legs stronger. Variations of the bodyweight lunge include holding dumbbells, adding bicep curls, resistance bands or overhead presses.

HOW TO DO A LUNGE EXERCISE

- Stand straight, with your shoulders relaxed and feet in line with the hips.
- Take one big step forward, shifting your bodyweight over that foot.
- Bring your rear foot backward, bending the ankle and balancing on your toes
- Distribute your weight evenly between the two legs. Put your hands on your hips or out in front of you for stability.
- Bend your knees, lowering your body until the back shin is parallel to the floor and the front shin is vertical. Your front leg should be bent about 90 degrees.
- Bring yourself back up by driving your front heel into the ground while slowly extending your leg.

BODYWEIGHT SQUAT

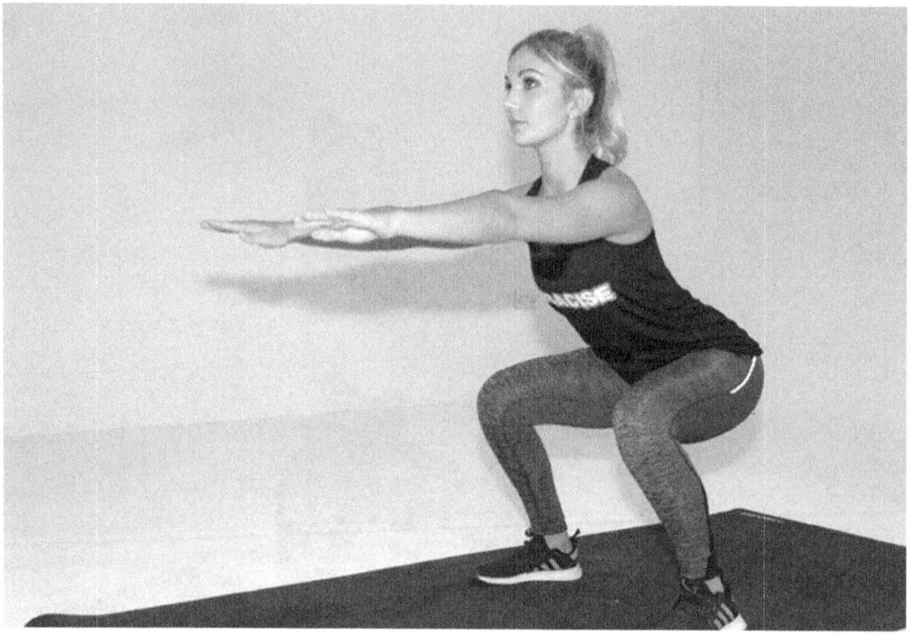

The squat is a compound exercise for the lower body that primarily trains your quadriceps and glutes. Performing the squat can lead to stronger bones, ligaments, and tendons. Squats are one of the most popular leg exercises.

Squats are very versatile as they can be done anywhere. You can also multitask by adding another exercise to make them harder, such as Overhead Power Press or Bicep Curls. Once the standard bodyweight squat becomes too easy for you, there are a multitude of variations. Adding weight is very common for both bodybuilders and powerlifters, or if you want to keep the squat a bodyweight exercise, you could try jumping squats.

HOW TO DO A BODYWEIGHT SQUAT

- Stand with your head facing forward, keeping your shoulders straight and chest held up and out.
- Make sure your feet are shoulder-width apart, with toes pointed slightly outwards and glutes squeezed.
- Sit back and down, like you're sitting on an invisible chair. Keep your body square with your feet.
- As you descend, extend your arms in front of you to help maintain balance.
- Bring your thighs parallel to the floor, or as low as you can. Make sure your heels remain flat by pushing your weight backward.
- Push through your heels to bring yourself up to the starting position.

Exercise Name	Main Muscle worked	Compound/Isolation	Equipment needed
Star Jump	Quadriceps	Compound	Bodyweight
Jumping Jack	Quadriceps	Compound	Bodyweight
Crab Walk	Quadriceps	Compound	Bodyweight
Clock Lunge	Quadriceps	Compound	Bodyweight
Butt Kick	Quadriceps	Compound	Bodyweight
Frog Jump	Quadriceps	Compound	Bodyweight
Burpee Box Jump	Quadriceps	Compound	Box, step
Jumping Jacks	Quadriceps	Compound	Bodyweight
Burpee	Quadriceps	Compound	Bodyweight
Mountain Climber	Quadriceps	Compound	Bodyweight
Jumping Lunge	Quadriceps	Compound	Bodyweight
Jump Squat	Quadriceps	Compound	Bodyweight
Bench Hop-Over	Quadriceps	Compound	Bodyweight
Ski Jump	Quadriceps	Compound	Bodyweight

You can find out more about these other quadricep exercises via the website: www.urbacise.com/exercises

BULGARIAN SPLIT SQUAT

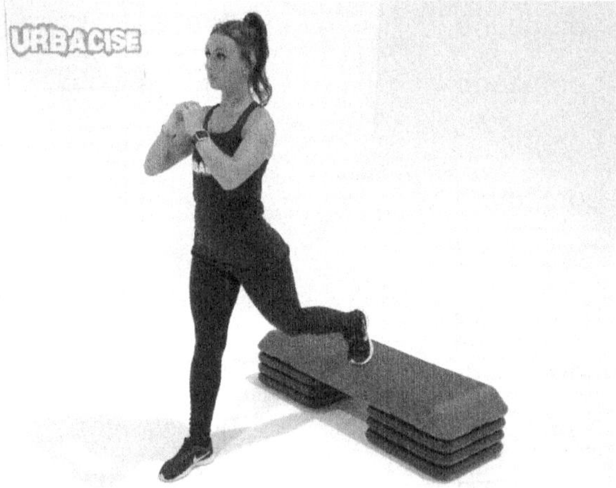

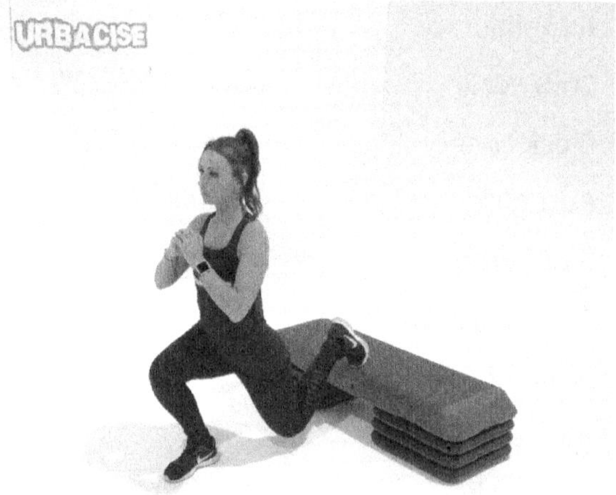

The Bulgarian split squat exercise strengthens the upper leg, helping to give extra support for the spine. This is a single leg advanced variation of the regular squat, targeting your glutes and quadriceps, with your hamstrings and calves acting as stabilizers. This exercise is very easy to perform, since the only equipment you need is a step and/or a box. When this exercise becomes too easy, you can add weight by holding a kettlebell or dumbbells by your side or increase the height of the step/box.

HOW TO DO A BULGARIAN SPLIT SQUAT EXERCISE

- Stand up straight with a step or box placed behind you.
- Like a reverse lunge, extend one leg backward, resting your toe on top of the step.
- Your front leg should be supporting most of your bodyweight, with your back leg and arms helping with balance.
- Bend your front knee, slowly squatting down until you reach a 90 degree angle.
- Your back knee should now be hovering slightly above the floor.
- You should feel a stretch in your glutes. If you don't, add weight or increase the height of the step.
- Return to the upper position by pushing through your heel while extending your front leg.

BARBELL HIP THRUST

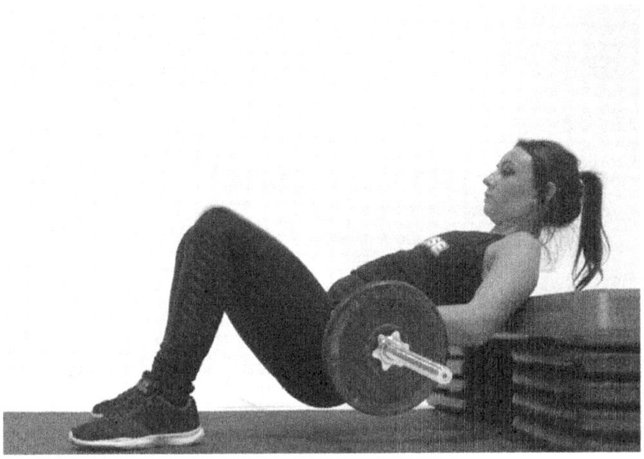
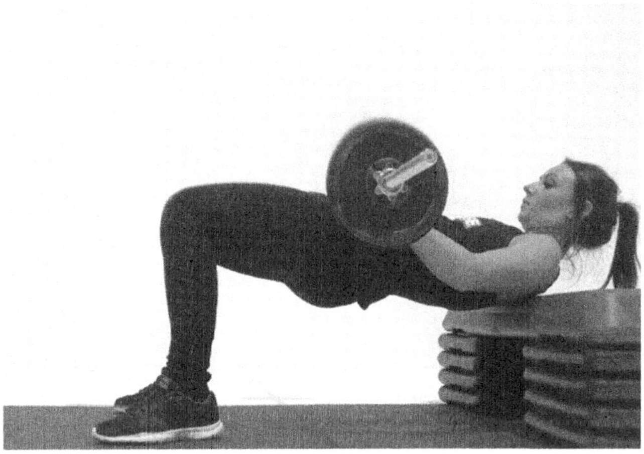

The barbell hip thrust exercise targets the glutes and helps strengthen the lower body. For an easier variation, you can use only your bodyweight or try glute bridges. To make this exercise more challenging, simply add more weight.

HOW TO DO A BARBELL HIP THRUST EXERCISE

- Sit on the floor with your legs stretched out in front of you. Place a barbell across your hips and a step, box or bench behind you.
- Lean backward, bringing your knees in, keeping them shoulder-width apart and in line with your toes. Both your knees and toes should be pointed slightly outward.
- The step should now be supporting your back, just below the shoulder blades.
- Thrust your hips upwards, bringing the barbell up with you.
- Pause when your knees are 90 degrees and your back is parallel to your thighs. Be careful not to overextend your spine. Look down your body towards the barbell or keep your head in a neutral position.
- When you feel the contraction in your glutes, slowly lower your hips back down.

MORE EXERCISES FOR YOUR GLUTES

Exercise Name	Main Muscle worked	Compound/Isolation	Equipment needed
Fire Hydrant	Glutes	Isolation	Bodyweight
Kickbacks	Glutes	Isolation	Bodyweight
Barbell Hip Thrust	Glutes	Isolation	Barbell
Bird Dog	Glutes	Compound	Bodyweight
Shoulder Bridge	Glutes	Isolation	Bodyweight
Flutter Kick	Glutes	Isolation	Bodyweight
Donkey Kick	Glutes	Isolation	Bodyweight
Bridge	Glutes	Isolation	Bodyweight

You can find out more about these other glute exercises via the website: www.urbacise.com/exercises

HAMSTRING EXERCISES

DEADLIFT

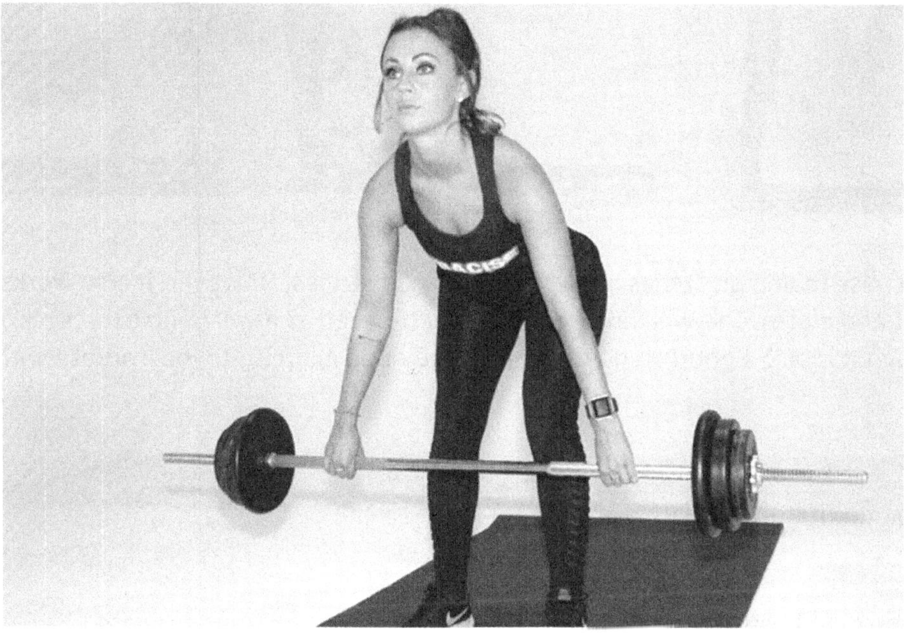

Deadlifts are another popular compound exercise. You might remember reading earlier that deadlifts exercise both your back and hamstrings, so you could either perform this exercise on your upper, lower or pull split day. This exercise also targets your quadriceps and glutes. Deadlifts are good for strength training and even help to improve your grip strength. The only equipment needed for a deadlift is a barbell. However, before loading the barbell with a heavy load, please remember how easy it Is to injure yourself without correct form.

HOW TO DO A DEADLIFT

- Stand with your feet shoulder-width apart with the barbell on the floor in front of you.
- Squat down to pick up the bar, keeping your hands about shoulder-width apart as well. Hold the bar with an overhand grip.
- Begin to stand, gripping the barbell tightly.
- Try to keep the bar as close to your legs as possible when coming up, as if you were sliding the bar up your body.
- Once you are fully standing, engage your glutes so your hips are pushed slightly forward Be careful not to bend your back too much.
- To finish the exercise, lower yourself back down again. This represents one repetition.

WALKOUT

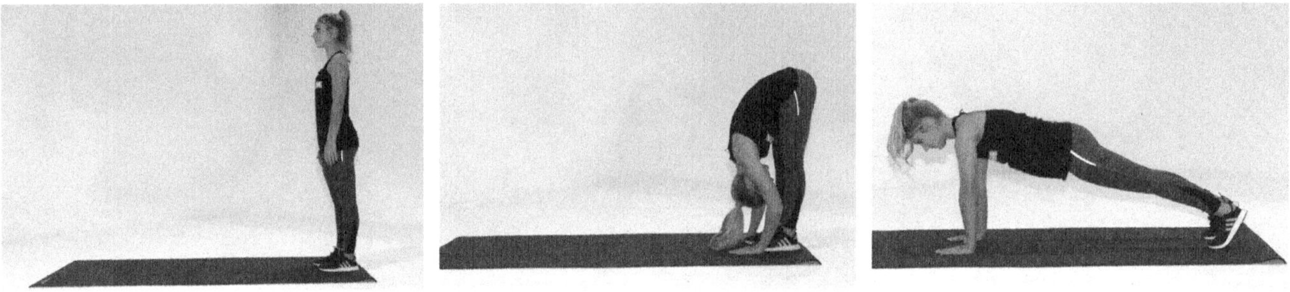

The walkout exercise mainly stretches and works your hamstrings. However, it also works your core, shoulders, chest and glutes. The walkout is normally performed as a warm-up exercise prior to your main workout, although it is also a good stand-alone exercise or an exercise to incorporate within your active rest.

HOW TO DO A WALKOUT EXERCISE

- Stand up straight with your feet hip-width apart and toes pointing forward.
- Bend at the hips, keeping your legs as straight as possible. Reach down and place both hands on the floor.
- With your feet fixed, walk your hands out in front of you. You should feel a stretch in your hamstrings.
- Keep walking your hands out until your body is in the upper push-up position, with hands directly below the shoulders.
- Keep your arms fully extended and hold for a moment.
- Now, walk your hands back toward your feet. Remember, try not to bend your legs.
- Stand up straight to finish the move.

MORE EXERCISES FOR YOUR HAMSTRINGS

Exercise Name	Main Muscle worked	Compound/Isolation	Equipment needed
Single Leg Deadlift	Hamstrings	Compound	Barbell
Stiff-Legged Deadlift	Hamstrings	Compound	Barbell
Tuck Jump	Hamstrings	Compound	Bodyweight
Box Jumps	Hamstrings	Compound	Box, Step
Stability Ball Hamstring Curl	Hamstrings	Isolation	Stability Ball

You can find out more about these other hamstring exercises via the website: www.urbacise.com/exercises

BACK EXERCISES

PULL-UP

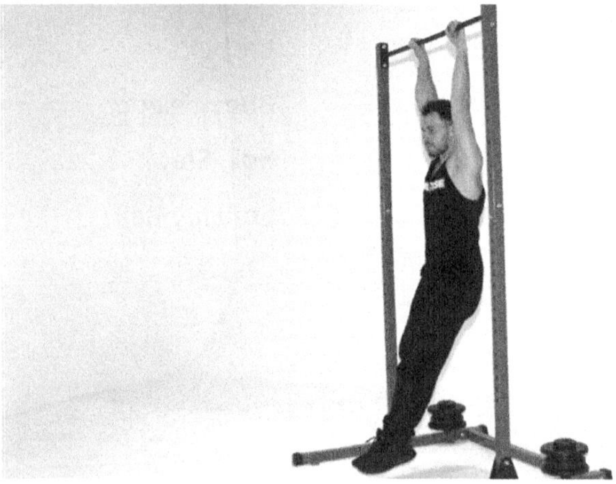 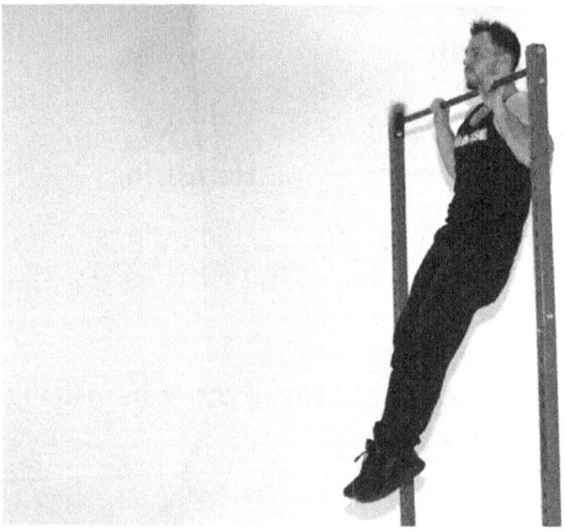

The pull-up exercise mainly targets your back and biceps. Your abs are also used to stabilize your body. The pull-up is one of the most popular bodyweight compound exercises and is a foundation for more advanced calisthenics exercises, such as the muscle-up.

HOW TO DO A PULL-UP EXERCISE

- Grab the pull-up bar with an overhand grip. Your hands should be shoulder-width apart or slightly wider.
- Take your feet off the floor and hang, with your arms straight and shoulder blades down.
- As you pull yourself up, squeeze your shoulder blades together.
- Keep the rest of your body straight by engaging your core. Don't swing, kick or use momentum to aid you.
- When your chin is above the bar, hold for a moment, before slowly lowering yourself back down.
- Fully extend your arms to finish the move, ensuring you have used your full range of motion.

RENEGADE ROWS

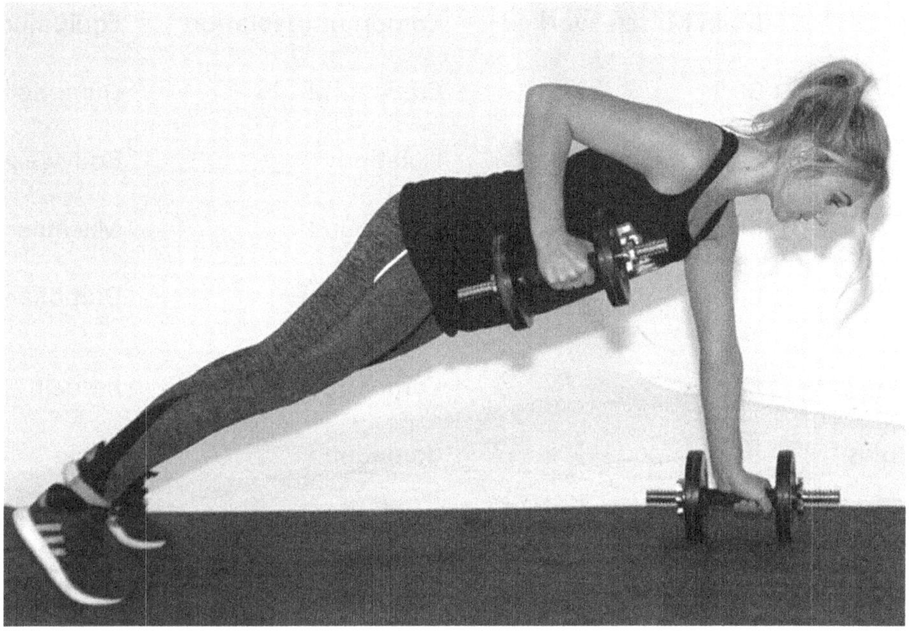

The Renegade Row is another compound exercise that primarily works your back muscles. However, it also exercises your chest, shoulders, triceps, biceps, and core. This is a great exercise to incorporate with either your upper body workout, pull split or within your circuit training (We'll be discussing circuit training later). The only equipment needed for this exercise is a pair of dumbbells. If you are not confident balancing on dumbbells (as they tend to roll outwards), then you can either purchase or find some square dumbbells, which would offer more stability, or use a single weight plate.

HOW TO DO A RENEGADE ROW

- Begin in the upper push-up position, with a dumbbell in each hand. Make sure your body is straight. Avoid putting your backside in the air or sagging your hips downward.
- Pull one dumbbell upwards towards your chest, beginning to bend your arm until your elbow passes your upper back. Try to avoid rotating your hips.
- Lower the dumbbell back down to the ground.
- Repeat this movement with the opposite arm. This would be one repetition.

Exercise Name	Main Muscle worked	Compound/Isolation	Equipment needed
Man Maker	Back	Compound	Dumbbell
Superman	Back	Isolation	Bodyweight
Lat Pulldown	Back	Compound	Machine
Single Arm Dumbbell Row	Back	Isolation	Dumbbell
Bent Over Barbell Row	Back	Compound	Barbell
Seated Cable Rows	Back	Compound	Cable
Inverted Rows	Back	Compound	Bodyweight
Renegade Rows	Back	Compound	Dumbbell
Plyometric Pull-up	Back	Compound	Bodyweight
Inverted Row	Back	Compound	Bodyweight

You can find out more about these other back exercises via the website: www.urbacise.com/exercises

CHEST EXERCISES

PUSH-UP

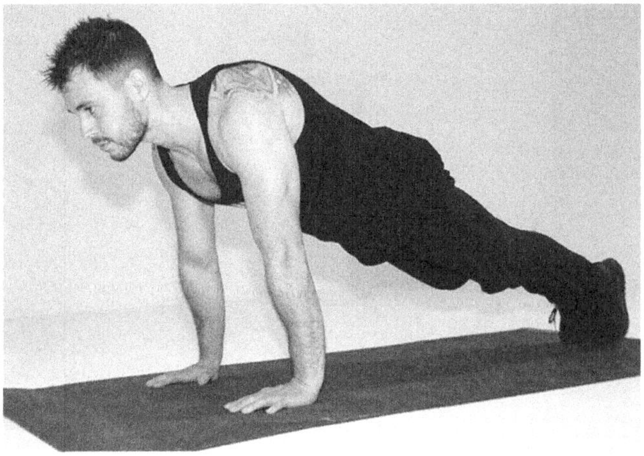

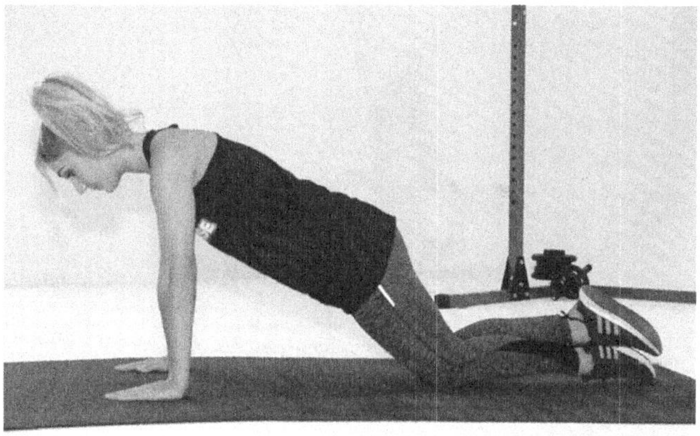

The push-up exercise mainly targets your chest, shoulders, triceps, and abs. If you find this variation too challenging, perform the exercise on your knees. To make the push up even harder, elevate your legs by placing your feet on a raised surface.

No equipment is needed for a push-up, so you can do these anywhere.

HOW TO DO A PUSH-UP EXERCISE

- Squat down, placing your hands on the floor.
- Walk your hands out in front of you.
- Stop when your body is straight, and arms fully extended. Your hands should be in line with your shoulders.
- Slowly lower your body toward the ground. This will force your shoulder blades together.
- When your elbows are bent 90 degrees, pause for a moment, keeping your abs engaged and ensuring your body is straight.
- Come back up by pushing against the floor and extending your arms.

FRONT DIP

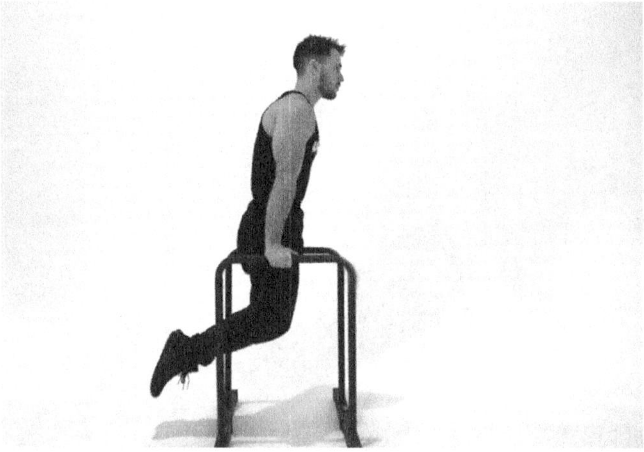
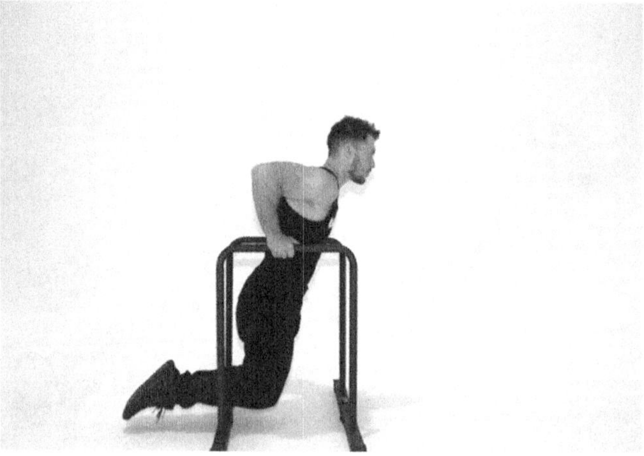

The front dip is a compound push exercise that mainly works your chest and triceps, but also works your shoulders and back. It's called the front dip because you are holding the bars in front of your chest as opposed to behind as you would in a tricep box dip, for example.

Front dips are simple to perform as they do not require very much equipment. Dip bars are standard in health clubs and most gyms. You can even do them at home by supporting your weight between two sturdy objects.

HOW TO DO A FRONT DIP

- Hold the parallel bars with straight arms. Pull your feet up off the ground and support your bodyweight.
- Keep your shoulders back and engage your abs.
- For extra stability, cross your legs behind you. Remember to keep looking forward with your head up.
- As you lower yourself down, keep your chest slightly forward with your elbows behind. Avoid widening your elbows or allowing them to touch your torso.
- Keep lowering yourself down until your arms are at least at a 90 degree angle. If you have more strength and a greater range of motion, you can go deeper.
- Now, push yourself back up to the starting position.

MORE EXERCISES FOR YOUR CHEST

Exercise Name	Main Muscle worked	Compound/Isolation	Equipment needed
Bench Press	Chest	Compound	Barbell
Diamond Push-Up	Chest	Isolation	Bodyweight
Chest Throw	Chest	Compound	Medicine ball
Bench Press	Chest	Compound	Barbell
Tiger Bend Push-up	Chest	Compound	Bodyweight
Muay Thai Push-Up	Chest	Compound	Bodyweight
Archer Push-Up	Chest	Compound	Bodyweight
Elephant Stand	Chest	Compound	Bodyweight
Plyometric Bench Press	Chest	Compound	Barbell
Medicine Ball Push Up	Chest	Compound	Medicine ball
Superman Push-up	Chest	Compound	Bodyweight
Decline Push-Up	Chest	Compound	Box, Step
Clapping Dip	Chest	Compound	Bodyweight

You can find out more about these other chest exercises via the website: www.urbacise.com/exercises

AB EXERCISES

PLANK

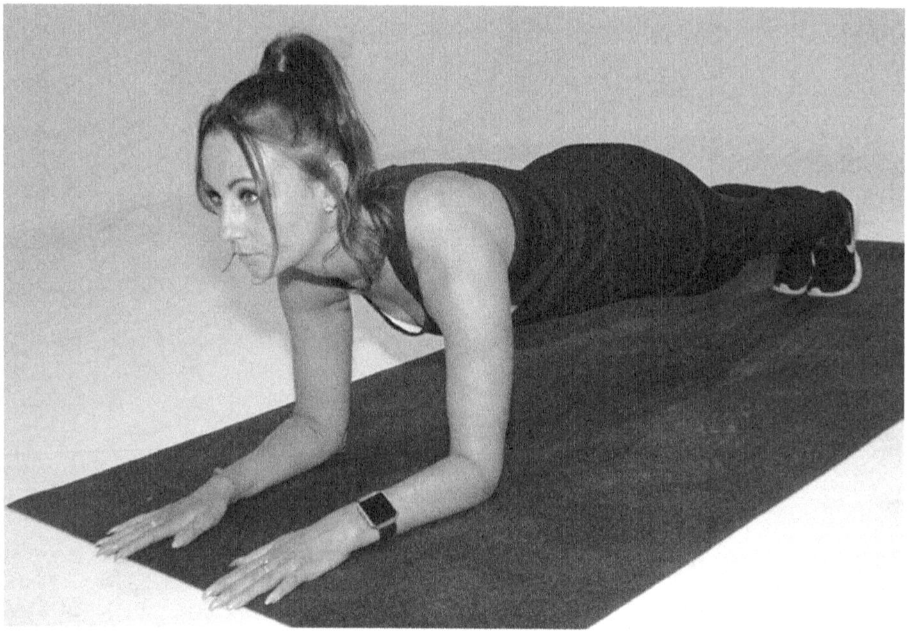

The front plank exercise is useful for improving balance, stability, and posture. It strengthens your whole core, including your back, glutes, shoulders, triceps, and hamstrings.

HOW TO DO A FRONT PLANK EXERCISE

- Lay on the floor. Put your forearms out in front of you. Your elbows should be by your side, directly under your shoulders. Your palms should be down, fingers facing forward. Your legs should be straight with your feet close together.
- Engage your core muscles. While keeping your body rigid, slowly lift your stomach and thighs off the floor.
- Your toes and forearms are now supporting all your bodyweight. Bend your ankles 90 degrees.
- Breathe normally and hold your position.
- Keep your body straight in a neutral position. Don't let your lower back arch or have your hips too high.

Place your feet wider apart if this move is too challenging. Once you can hold it for over a minute, consider progressing to a more advanced variation, such as lifting one foot off the floor.

RUSSIAN TWIST

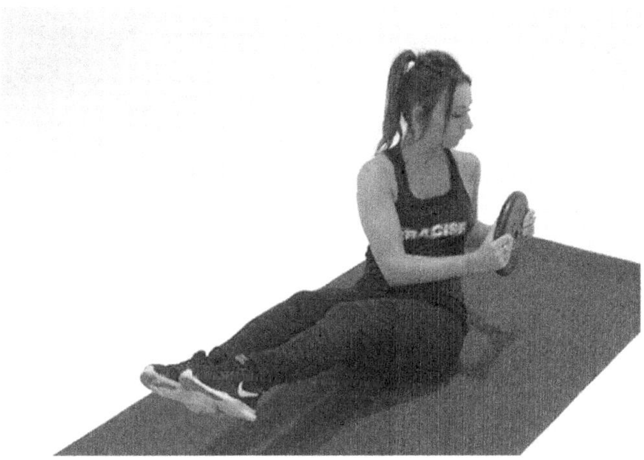

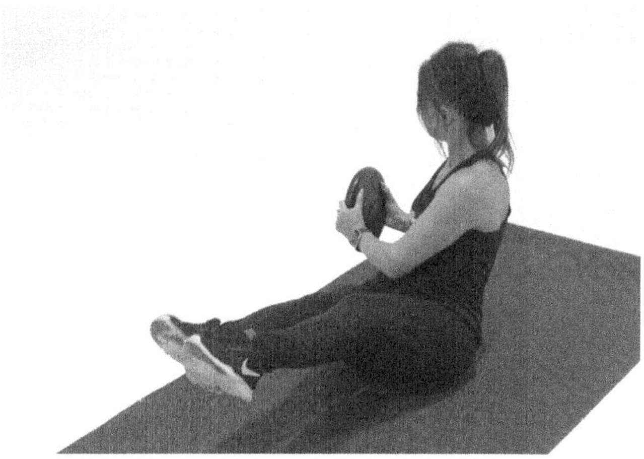

Russian twists target your abdominal muscles, including your obliques. No equipment is required to perform this exercise, however, if you want more of a challenge, you can use a weight.

HOW TO DO A RUSSIAN TWIST EXERCISE

- Sit on the floor with your legs in front of you, bending your knees slightly.
- Hold the weight in front of your chest and lean back to engage your core.
- Leading with your hips, twist your upper torso as far as you can to one side.
- Hold the weight fixed in front of your chest.
- Once you have reached maximum rotation, twist your torso to the other side

For more of a challenge, take your feet off the floor, and straighten your legs.

Exercise Name	Main Muscle worked	Compound/Isolation	Equipment needed
V-Sit	Core	Compound	Bodyweight
Sit-Up	Core	Compound	Bodyweight
Ab Crunches	Core	Compound	Bodyweight
Jackknife	Core	Compound	Bodyweight
Kneeling walkout	Core	Compound	Bodyweight
Russian Twist	Core	Compound	Bodyweight
Side Plank	Core	Compound	Bodyweight
Plank	Core	Compound	Bodyweight
Dead Bug	Core	Compound	Bodyweight
Plank to Push-Up	Core	Compound	Bodyweight
Bicycles	Core	Compound	Bodyweight
Scissor Kicks	Core	Isolation	Bodyweight
Cable Crunches	Core	Compound	Cable
Hanging Windshield Wiper	Core	Compound	Bodyweight
Leg Raises	Core	Compound	Bodyweight

You can find out more about these other core exercises via the website: www.urbacise.com/exercises

SHOULDER EXERCISES

MILITARY PRESS

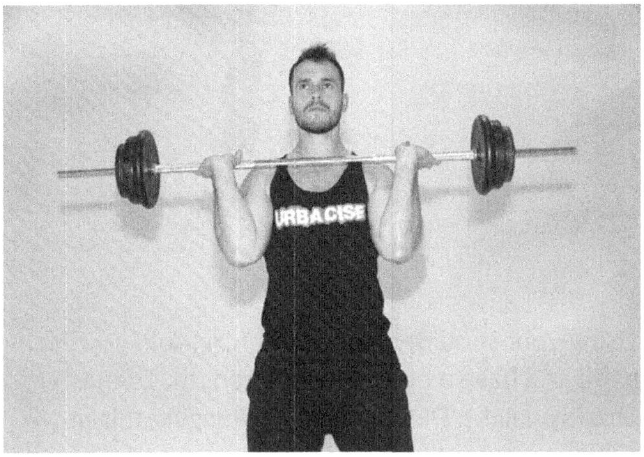

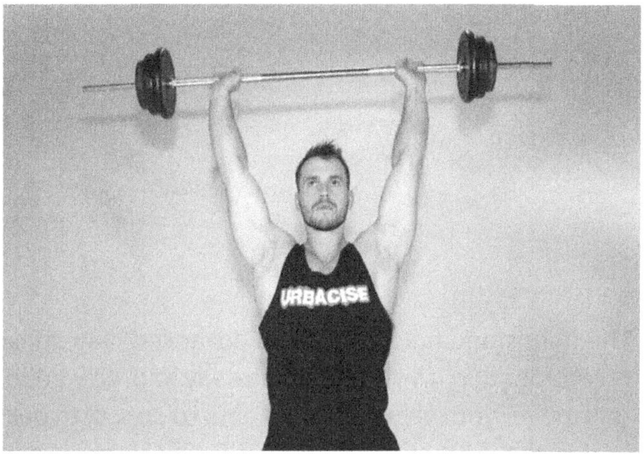

The military press is very popular with both bodybuilders and powerlifters. It's a compound upper body push exercise that works your shoulders, back, triceps, biceps, and chest. Again, with this exercise, it's very easy to injure yourself if you use too heavy a weight, so it's strongly recommended you warm up correctly and use correct form.

This exercise is typically performed with a barbell, so you can lift a heavier load. However, it can also be performed with dumbbells. The difference between the military press and power press is that with the military press you keep your legs straight. This prevents you from using the bounce you'd get if you were to bend your legs in the lower phase. Therefore, the military press is a lot harder than a power press.

To be able to lift the maximum amount of weight above your head, you should ideally use a squat rack, with the barbell already near shoulder height. This saves you from having to bend over to pick it up and possibly straining your back.

HOW TO DO A MILITARY PRESS

- Feet should be shoulder-width apart. Your hand grip should also be shoulder-width apart.
- Move your chest under the bar, lifting the bar slightly so it is free of the rack. Take a step backward.
- Keep your legs straight (don't bend them, as that would be a different move) then push the bar upwards, above your head and lock out your arms.
- After you have locked out, simply bring the barbell back down to shoulder height. The slower and more controlled you can do this, the more time you have under tension, which improves muscle growth. This would be one repetition.

HANDSTAND WALL HOLD

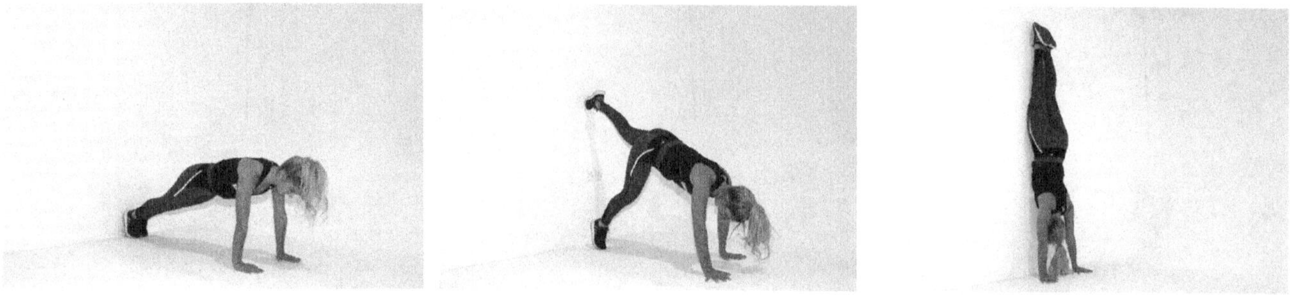

The handstand hold is quite an advanced way of exercising your shoulders. It is therefore not recommended if you are not already in pretty good shape and have a high level of strength. To master this move, you will need to be able to support your full bodyweight. Despite how challenging this move is, it is also a lot of fun and great for adding variation to your workout programs. Not many people in the gym seem to utilize this move.

HOW TO DO A HANDSTAND HOLD

- Start in the upper push-up position with your feet against a wall.
- Lift one leg and place it higher up the wall, and start walking your hands in towards the wall. Once you have both feet on the wall, you must be able to support your bodyweight
- Keep walking your hands and feet in until you're in a handstand.
- The closer you can get your hands to the wall, the harder this move will be. Once you have your hands as close as possible, hold the position.
- While in the handstand, try and keep your legs together. Make sure your body is straight and point your toes (this will help straighten your legs).

MORE EXERCISES FOR YOUR SHOULDERS

Exercise Name	Main Muscle worked	Compound/Isolation	Equipment needed
Lateral Raise	Shoulders	Isolation	Dumbbell
Military Press	Shoulders	Compound	Barbell
Clean and Press	Shoulders	Compound	Barbell
Handstand Wall Walk	Shoulders	Compound	Bodyweight
Handstand Push-Up	Shoulders	Compound	Bodyweight
Tuck Planche	Shoulders	Compound	Bodyweight
Pike Push-Up	Shoulders, Abs	Compound	Bodyweight
Handstand	Shoulders, Abs	Compound	Bodyweight

You can find out more about these other shoulder exercises via the website:
www.urbacise.com/exercises

CALF EXERCISES

STANDING CALF RAISE

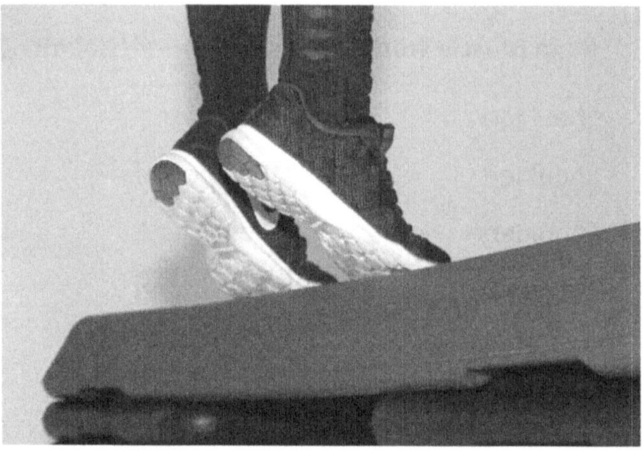

Calf raises are the most popular isolation exercise, designed to strengthen your calf muscles and improve your ankle strength and stability. This exercise can prevent injury: The stronger your calves are, the less likely they are to tear if you have a nasty fall. Strengthening these muscles can also really help improve your running and thereby your endurance in general.

HOW TO DO A STANDING CALF RAISE

- Stand on a raised surface (such as a weight plate or a pile of sturdy books) and have the ball of your feet on the edge of the raised surface with your heels overhanging. If you are not comfortable balancing in this position, move the raised surface next to a wall for extra support.
- With your heels overhanging, simply raise them up as high as possible, keeping your body straight.
- Once you have raised your heels as high as you are able, lower them back down. Your heels should surpass the bottom of the raised surface and you should feel the stretch in your calves.

MORE EXERCISES FOR YOUR CALVES

Exercise Name	Main Muscle worked	Compound/Isolation	Equipment needed
Seated Calf Raise	Calves	Isolation	Dumbbell
Standing Calf Raise	Calves	Isolation	dumbbell

You can find out more about these other calf exercises via the website: www.urbacise.com/exercises

TRICEP EXERCISES

TRICEPS BENCH DIP

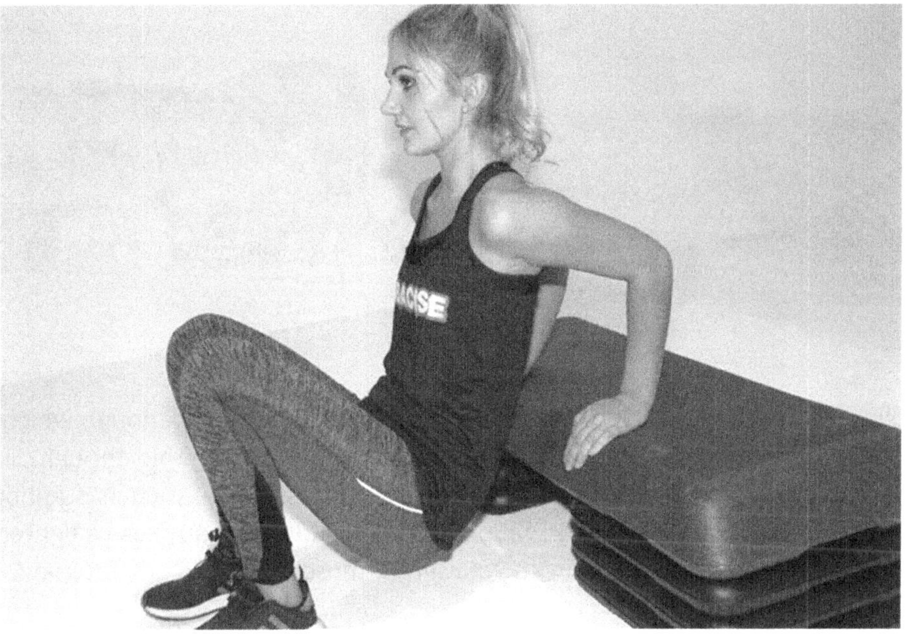

Tricep bench dips mainly target your triceps and chest as well as work your core.

HOW TO DO THE TRICEP BENCH DIP EXERCISE

- Sit on a bench or step, placing your hands next to your hips with your palms facing downward.
- Slide your bum off the front of the bench and support your bodyweight through your arms and legs.
- Bend your knees and have your arms fully extended.
- Slowly bend at the elbow and lower yourself toward the floor. Keep your back close to the bench.
- When your elbows are at 90 degrees, pause for a moment.
- Come back up by pushing against the bench and extending your arms.

For a harder variation try straightening your legs OR bring one foot up off the floor.

SKULL CRUSHERS

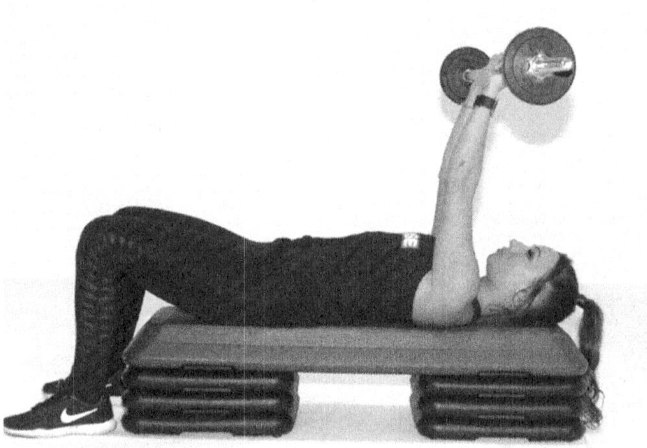

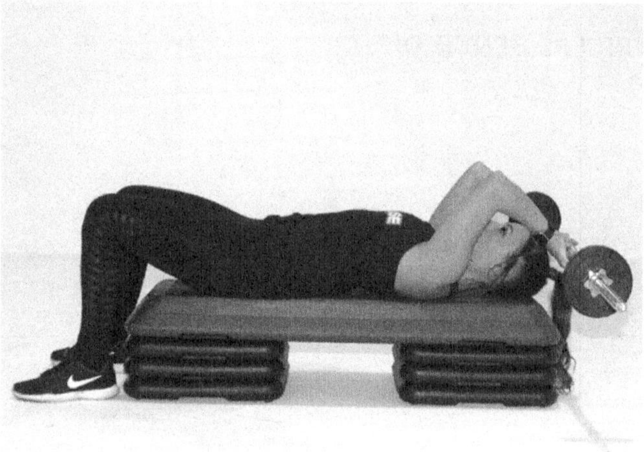

As the name implies, this exercise can be very dangerous and given a heavy enough weight the name of the exercise can probably come true. Don't let the name put you off trying this, though. Skull Crushers work your triceps and can be performed with various means of resistance, such as dumbbells, barbells and resistance bands. Skull Crushers are an isolation exercise, and you should use a lighter weight as you normally do these after compound exercises, so your larger muscles are already fatigued.

HOW TO DO THE SKULL CRUSHER EXERCISE

- Pick up the barbell using a narrow grip, slightly less than shoulder-width apart. Lay on the bench or step, bending your legs at 90 degrees and keeping your feet flat on the floor.
- Hold the barbell above your chest.
- Angle your upper arms towards your ears so the barbell is on a tilt while bending at the elbows. This will bring the barbell down past the top of your head.
- Keep your elbows pointing upwards, towards the ceiling. Make sure they are in tight; don't let them flare out to the sides.
- When your arms bend to roughly 90 degrees, slowly push the barbell back up to the starting position.

MORE EXERCISES FOR YOUR TRICEPS

Exercise Name	Main Muscle worked	Compound/Isolation	Equipment needed
Triceps Extension	Triceps	Compound	Dumbbells
Skull Crushers	Triceps	Isolation	Barbell
Elbow Dip	Triceps	Compound	Bodyweight
Triceps Bench Dip	Triceps	Compound	Bodyweight
Front Dip	Triceps, Chest	Compound	Bodyweight

You can find out more about these other exercises for your triceps via the website: www.urbacise.com/exercises

BICEP EXERCISES

BARBELL CURL

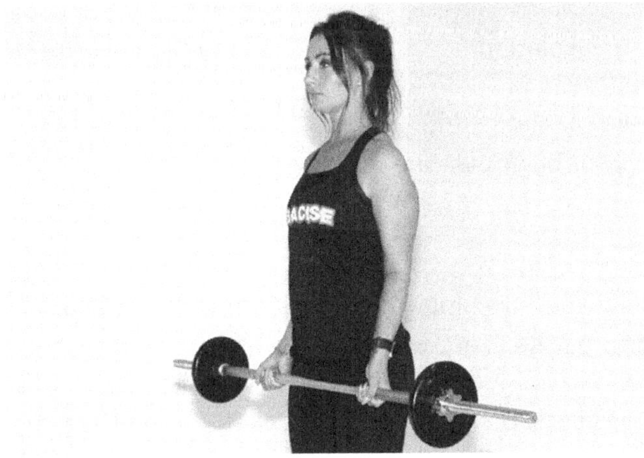

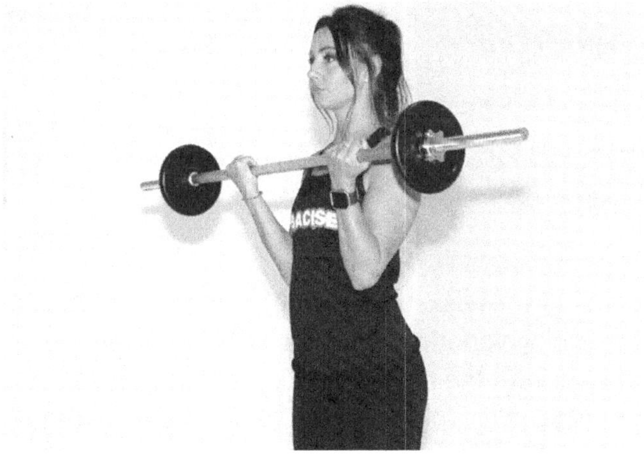

Barbell curls are a favorite isolation exercise for the biceps. You can use various equipment to train your biceps, though, including resistance bands and dumbbells. This exercise is great if you want to achieve proportionately bigger biceps or if you have developed muscle imbalances.

HOW TO DO A BARBELL CURL EXERCISE

- With your feet shoulder-width apart, squat down.
- Grip the barbell with an underhand grip.
- Extend your legs, bringing the barbell up with you. With your arms slightly bent and elbows tucked in by your side, rest the bar against your pelvis.
- Keep your posture straight and upright.
- Slowly bring the barbell up toward your chest, keeping your elbows locked in place.
- Squeeze your biceps when the bar approaches your chest.
- Slowly lower the barbell back down. Don't try to use momentum to aid you in any way; keep the movements smooth and controlled.

MORE EXERCISES FOR YOUR BICEPS

Exercise Name	**Main Muscle worked**	**Compound/Isolation**	**Equipment needed**
Stair Climb with Bicep Curl	Bicep	Compound	Dumbbell
Bicep Curl	Bicep	Isolation	Dumbbell
Barbell Curl	Biceps	Isolation	Barbell

You can find out more about these other exercises for your biceps via the website: www.urbacise.com/exercises

Some of these exercises will be less efficient than others when training your muscles, but they are good for adding variation. The most efficient exercise tends to be the exercise that allows you to train that muscle with the most possible weight. Don't worry if you're not looking to lift heavy weights, the principle still applies. The well-known exercises such as squats, bench press and deadlifts are still ideal.

Experiment with some of the exercises on the list and don't forget you can learn more about all the exercises via the Urbacise website through our exercise database www.urbacise.com/exercises.

BARBELL VS DUMBBELL

Have you ever wondered if it's best to do an exercise with a barbell or a dumbbell?

Dumbbells give you a better range of motion (ROM), and if you are using them in an upper body exercise such as the chest press, they allow for a more natural movement. They also let you go "deeper" with your movements, so you put the muscle under more stress. With the barbell, however, you can do unilateral movements, which means there are fewer imbalances and you develop independent motion control. With a barbell chest press, you can lift heavier weights, since not as much stability is needed. If you are new to weightlifting it is recommended that you stick with the barbell bench press for now as it's easier to injure yourself using dumbbells.

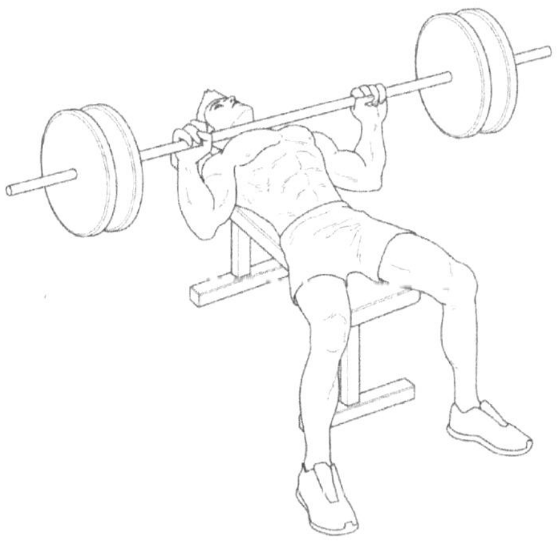

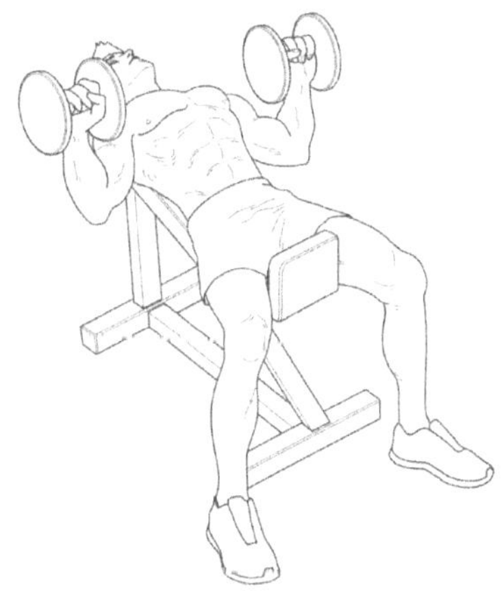

Some exercises are more suited to barbells than dumbbells, especially when using weight as an aid to increase the difficulty of an exercise. An example is weighted squats, where you would put yourself at more risk of getting injured if you attempted heavy squats using dumbbells.

When deciding whether to perform an exercise with a barbell or a dumbbell, ask yourself whether using a dumbbell would increase the range of motion for that exercise and seem like a more natural moment without it putting you at in any kind of risk or in an uncomfortable situation.

CHAPTER SIX: CHOOSE HOW MANY REPS TO DO

Now that you know what types of exercises to put into your exercise program and what order to put them in, you will want to determine how many reps of these exercises to do.

Terminology: Repetitions are simply the number of times you perform an exercise, abbreviated in the gym to "reps." For example, if you do two push-ups, that means you've effectively done two push-up reps.

The number of reps you should do per exercise depends entirely on your work out goals. Do you want more:

- **Power**? Perhaps you'd like to be more explosive if you're training for a sport such as long jump.
- **Strength**? If you're a powerlifter, you'll want to lift as much as possible.
- **Size?** Maybe you want to look more muscular for the sake of appearance, like a bodybuilder.
- **Aerobic exercise/Conditioning?** Many people want a healthier/more efficient body. This is also good if you're training for an event such as an obstacle race.

You should know that your body always adapts to best ensure your survival. Our body adapts to the pressures we put it under. If you struggle to do a necessary task and need to be stronger, doing that task repeatedly, will make you stronger. With that in mind, you need to know your goal in order to determine the best way to train your muscles towards achieving it.

For more information, please see the appendices:

How do muscles grow and recover? (Page 104)

How does working out build muscle? (Page 106)

If you're training for size, strength or power (really, anything other than fitness), you should ideally know your "one-rep max" of each exercise you plan to do. We will use a percentage of this to help determine the number of reps you perform.

Figure 32: Weighted Barbell Squat (A popular one-rep max exercise)

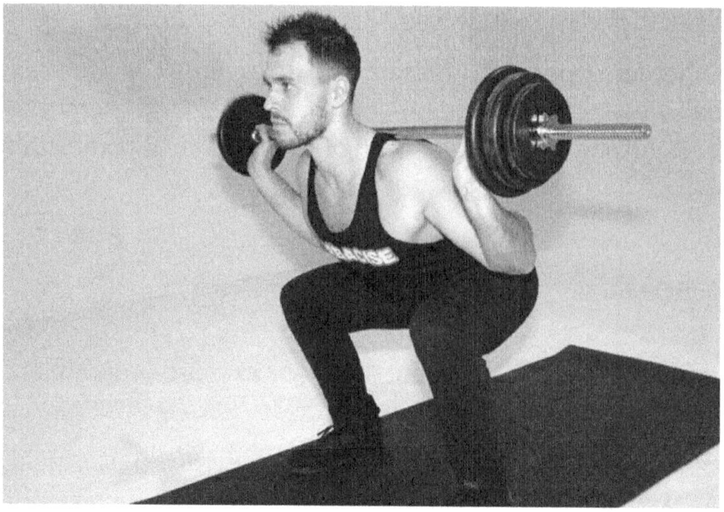

When trying out your one rep max for any exercise, make sure you have someone to help you (this person is called a spotter). This type of lift can be very dangerous, and it's easy to injure yourself if you lift too heavy a weight. It's important that you warm up before lifting heavy weights as well. We'll be discussing this a little later. Once you've worked out your one rep max you can then roughly determine the amount of weight needed for the various number of reps to help reach your goal.

THE OPTIMAL NUMBER OF REPS DEPENDING ON YOUR FITNESS GOALS:

- **Power** = 2 to 5 reps per set
- **Strength** = 6 to 8 reps per set
- **Size** = 8 to 12 reps per set
- **Aerobic exercise/Fitness** = More than 12 reps per set

For more information please see appendices: **Dense muscles vs. Big muscles (Page 107)**

Figure 33: Military Press (Upper hold)

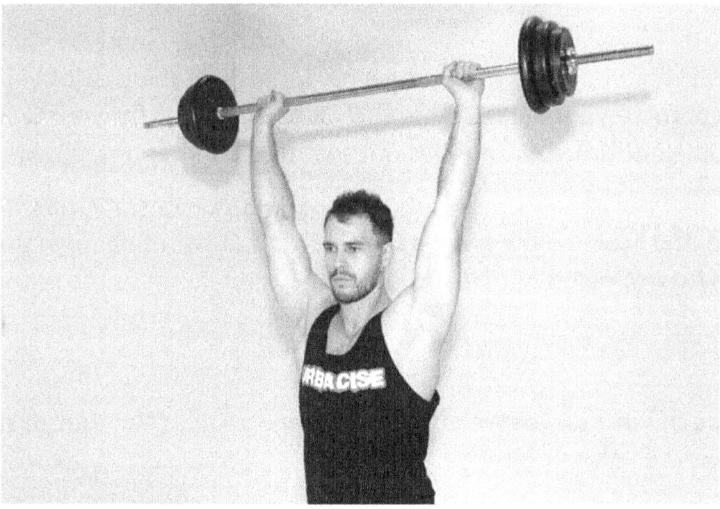

Let's take the military press as an example exercise (***Figure 33***). You can't just do 2 to 5 reps with any amount of weight and still build your power. If you can do more than 5 reps with the amount of weight you choose, then that weight is too light for you to achieve that goal efficiently. If you're training for power and you can do more than 5 military presses with the barbell, then you should add weight to the barbell until you can only do between 2 to 5 reps.

Here is a table that gives examples of what your weight might be (as a percentage of your one-rep max) for the number of reps that fall within your desired goal:

Number of repetitions	Percentage of one-rep max
1	100%
2	95%
3	93%
4	90%
5	87%
6	85%
7	83%
8	80%
9	77%
10	75%
11	70%
12	67%

START YOUR WORKOUT WITH A WARM-UP

It's recommended to base your warm-up weight on a percentage of the weight you intend to lift. The idea of warming up is to prepare yourself both mentally and physically for your workout (to prevent injury) but at the same time not tire your muscles out too much that you're unable to lift the desired amount.

With that in mind, the table below gives a safe method of warming up in preparation for any weightlifting. You start by warming up with just the bar and then increase the weight until you are close to your target weight.

Weight (As a percentage of your target weight)	Warm up Reps (Number of reps)
Just the bar	10 - 15
55 - 60%	8
70 - 75%	5
80 - 85%	3
90 - 95%	1

To avoid confusion, use these percentages as a guide as opposed to an absolute rule.

For more information please see appendices: **Dense muscle vs big muscles (Page 107)**

TIME UNDER TENSION

One of the best methods for maximizing the efficiency of your reps is by increasing the amount of 'time under tension.' Time under tension is the amount of time that a muscle is being strained. To get the most benefit from time under tension, you need to stay in control of your lift and focus on engaging the muscles you are targeting. Ideally, you want to maintain a consistent tempo during each repetition. Typically, the ideal tempo is approximately 3 seconds during the up phase and 3-4 seconds during the down phase of your lift. If possible, make sure that the eccentric part of your lift is equal to or longer than the concentric part of your lift. For those who don't know, the eccentric phase of your lift is when your muscles are lengthening under tension. For example, it's the downward movement during the bicep curl, bench press or squat. The concentric part of your lift is when your muscle shortens under tension, such as during the upward movement in a bicep curl.

CHAPTER SEVEN: CIRCUIT TRAINING

With circuit training, you can shorten your workouts and make them more exciting at the same time. You can either do circuit training based on the number of reps or a certain time duration.

WHAT IS CIRCUIT TRAINING?

Circuit training is where you complete several different exercises in quick succession with minimal rest. For instance, you might have four exercises:

- Squats x 10 reps OR 30 seconds
- Superman x 30 seconds
- Walkout x 10 reps OR 30 seconds
- Push-Ups x 10 reps OR 30 seconds

This would repeat for three rounds having a minute's rest between each round.

You would then rest for a minute after completing all the exercises before going again. This example uses only your bodyweight, but you could easily add weight or change this to just a particular body part.

If you've been reading carefully, you might be able to tell how I arrived at the above workout. I followed the upper/lower split and I alternated between front and back muscles. When you're structuring your circuit training, you can still follow the fundamentals we've mentioned in the previous pages.

Weighted circuit training allows you to complete more reps and more sets in a shorter amount of time. This not only means you burn more calories, but you increase your work capacity — the amount of stress and volume your muscles can handle. You'll also get more proficient in the exercises because you're practicing them more intensely. Remember, even if you are trying to complete a circuit as fast as you can, always make sure to focus on your form above anything else.

PROS OF CIRCUIT TRAINING

- Faster sessions and more efficient.
- Increases your work capacity.
- Burns more calories.
- Helps you to practice each movement under stress.
- Easily adaptable based upon what body part you want to focus on.
- Can be done weighted or unweighted.
- Some people find it more engaging than standard routines.
- Can combine cardio and resistance training into one.

CONS OF CIRCUIT TRAINING

- Not the best if your main focus is time under tension.
- Can result in injuries if you do not concentrate on form.
- Requires a base level of cardio performance (due to minimal rest).

Figure 34: Circuit Training Example

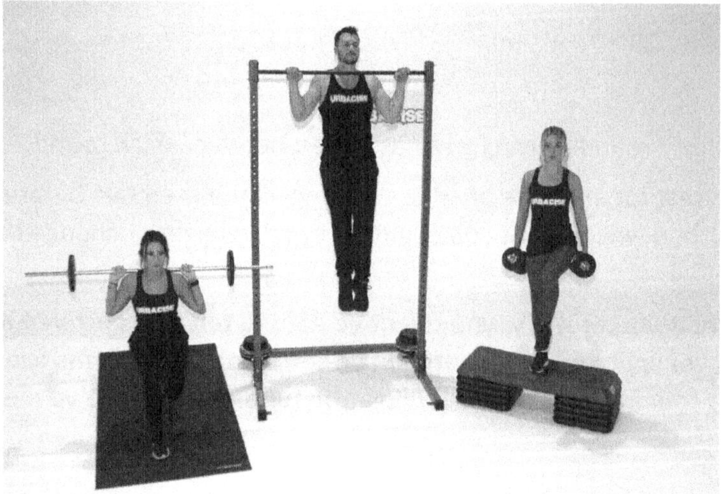

You don't have to use circuit training every single session but switching one or two of your weekly workouts over to a circuit can really help to keep things interesting. At the end of the day, the best workout routine will be the one that you enjoy the most and helps you progress towards your goals.

CHAPTER EIGHT: SHOULD YOU TRAIN UNTIL FAILURE?

When people are training to gain strength, many wonder if they should be training to failure. While some people argue that this training method will do nothing but cause injuries, others believe that it's the most effective way to build strong muscles. The key to getting the most benefit out of strength training, until you reach failure, is doing it properly.

Any time we take part in strength training, or any type of exercise for that matter, there is a risk of injury. However, most strength training injuries do not necessarily occur as a result of training to failure. Most injuries result from improper lifting techniques, bad form, and doing too much too soon. When you are training, there are different types of failure, including:

- **Tempo Failure -** This is when you begin to struggle to lift the weight or perform the reps at the same speed as you did when you first started your set.
- **Technique Failure -** This is when your form starts to suffer as you continue performing your reps.
- **Tolérance Failure -** This is best described as the burning sensation that you get in your muscles during your workout that makes it hard for you to keep going.

Figure 35: Renegade Rows

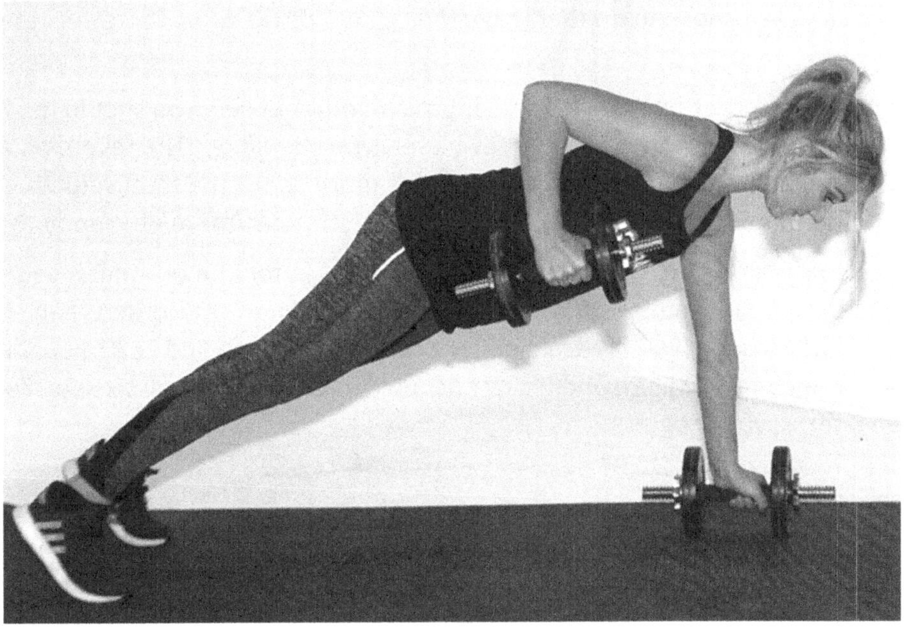

If you are doing your set and feeling a burning sensation in your muscles that causes you to slow down your pace while lifting, then you are experiencing tolerance and tempo failure. At that point, you are still doing useful reps that will be hugely beneficial to developing your overall strength. However, the moment you have to alter your form in order to perform your reps, you experience technique failure. In this case, technique failure is the only type of failure that puts you at risk of injury when strength training. As soon as you begin to experience technique failure, all the reps that follow are completely useless and do more harm than good.

So, if you are strength training and you "feel the burn", you can keep going for a few more reps — and doing so will help you get stronger over time. For example, if you struggled to do 16 bicep curls with a certain weight but managed to complete the set without compromising your form, you've achieved tolerance failure. Eventually, your body will adapt to the demand you place upon it and you will get to a point where you will be able to do 18 reps before you reach failure. Then, it will take 20 reps. After that, in order to get stronger, you will need to also progressively increase the weight. After a few months of consistent training, it may take you 20 reps of bicep curls with even more weight before you experience failure. Tempo failure is most useful for athletes who are training for explosive power. This type of training requires you to stop your set when you can no longer perform your reps at a certain speed.

Training to failure will help you gain strength provided that you use proper form when performing your reps. If you take adequate time to recover after your strength training session, your muscles will repair themselves and get stronger. Once you recover, it will take more weight or more reps to reach failure. Training to failure is an effective way to strength train if it's done correctly.

CHAPTER NINE: CHOOSE HOW MANY SETS TO DO

Now that you know how many reps you should do, we need to figure out how many sets you should do.

Terminology: A set is the number of cycles you do of that exercise. So, if I did 20 push-ups, 20 is the number of reps. If I then chose to do that three times, I would be doing three sets of push-ups, doing 20 reps each time.

There are many different opinions on the optimal number of sets you should do. As a general guide, the more reps you do of an exercise, the fewer sets you should do. The reverse is also true: The fewer reps you do, the more sets you should perform. It's more about the total volume. Ultimately, we're trying to tear our muscles, so they rebuild themselves stronger/more efficiently than before.

When this book refers to doing eight or more reps to train for size or fitness, you should do three sets or less. However, if you're training for power or strength and performing less than eight reps, you should be doing around six sets. If you're training for power or strength and you're unable to do six sets, this means you've hit technique failure and it's not necessary for you to do all six sets. You can add the additional sets on later as you progress.

Figure 36: Bent Over Barbell Row

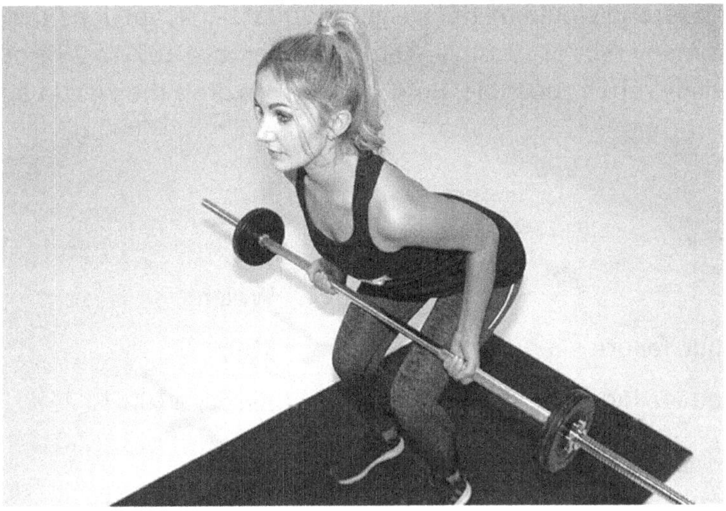

Popular types of sets:

- Straight sets
- Drop sets
- Pyramid sets
- Supersets

STRAIGHT SETS

Straight sets are the most common sort of set. They are simply when you do as many reps as you can, rest to let your body recover, and then do the same amount of reps (with the same amount of weight) again. These are very common and straightforward.

<u>Example</u>

Sets	Reps	Weight
#1	12	75% of one-rep max
#2	12	Same weight
#3	12	Same weight

DROP SETS

Drop sets allow you to extend your set. This helps to fatigue your muscle as much as possible by training until failure. An example exercise would be the weighted squat. First, you load the barbell with your desired weight and do as many reps as possible. You'd then remove 10% to 25% of the original weight, and immediately do as many reps as possible, until you need to drop the weight again.

Example

Set	**Reps**	**Weight**
#1	Until technique failure	100%
#2	Until technique failure	Remove 10% to 25%
#3	Until technique failure	Remove 10% to 25%
#4	Until technique failure	Remove 10% to 25%

ADVANTAGES OF DROP SETS

- Your muscles get even more fatigued. By decreasing the weight, you can do additional reps and help tear the muscle fibers more.
- Drop sets are used for building up strength and muscular endurance.

DISADVANTAGES OF DROP SETS

- Drop sets rapidly increase workload, so overtraining is more likely if used too often.
- You may need to acquire a spotter. If the initial set isn't taken to near failure, then the entire drop set is less effective.

PYRAMID SETS

Pyramid sets are where you start with a lighter weight, then increase the weight with each additional set until you reach the peak of the pyramid. You would then reverse and decrease the weight, normally back to the original weight. For instance, during the first set you would perform 10 reps with a certain weight; during the second set, you'd perform 8 sets with slightly more weight; and during the third set, you'd perform 6 sets with even more weight. Pyramid sets give you the chance to gradually warm up as you raise the intensity of your exercise.

Example

Set	Reps	Weight
#1	12	45%
#2	10	55%
#3	8	65%
#4	6	75%
#5	8	65%
#6	10	55%
#7	12	45%

ADVANTAGES OF PYRAMID SETS

- By using pyramid sets you can make your workouts more challenging. Pyramid sets are popular in CrossFit.
- These are great for power and strength training, often allowing you to do more reps than you would with normal straight sets.

DISADVANTAGES OF PYRAMID SETS

- It is not advisable to attempt to take your pyramid sets to the point of technical failure as it would be easy to injure yourself when doing so.

SUPERSETS

A **superset** is performed by combining two exercises back to back with no rest in between. The two exercises can be for the same muscle group, for opposing (antagonist) muscles, like biceps and triceps, or even non-competing muscle groups such as chest and calves.

There are three basic types of supersets:

- **Same muscle group:** The most commonly used superset involves combining two exercises for the same muscle group. One example for chest would be supersetting bench press with push-ups. Or for quadriceps, supersetting squats with leg press. This type of superset involves combining two compound exercises that will force your muscles to grow.

- **Antagonistic muscle supersets**: By supersetting opposing muscle groups together, you can train both harder — while one muscle is working, the opposite one is resting. Examples include biceps with triceps, chest with back, or hamstrings with quadriceps. This type of superset is also, an excellent approach for developing muscle balance. Hopefully you'll remember that many trainees overwork their pushing exercises like bench press while neglecting the pulling exercises like rows. By using antagonistic (or push-pull) supersets, you assure a good balance between opposing muscle groups.
- **Staggered sets**: Staggered sets train completely unrelated muscle groups, like shoulders and calves. An example would be to superset military press with calf raises. The main benefit of staggered sets is that they allow you to get your workout finished much quicker.

BENEFITS OF SUPERSETS

- **Supersets increase training intensity**. High-intensity muscle building techniques are often associated with forced reps, descending sets, and negative reps. Supersets are a simple method of increasing intensity because eliminating the rest between sets is hard work and overloads your body, especially if you're used to long rest periods. More work performed in less time equals increased intensity, and increased intensity leads to more muscle.
- **Supersets save you time.** Another advantage of supersetting is equal or better results in a shorter period. Eliminating the rest intervals between sets, when you would normally be inactive (and non-productive), you can finish your workout in half the time or perform more volume in the same amount of time.
- **Supersets can help you work around an injury.** When you do supersets, you must use lighter weights, especially on the second exercise, as you are eliminating the recovery between exercises. Supersets still allow you to overload a muscle with those lighter weights in a way that produces muscle growth because the work density is higher. Supersets also decrease joint stress and allow you to work around injuries with alternative exercises.
- **Supersets stimulate Growth Hormone (GH) production.** Supersets increase intensity and intensity stimulates lactic acid production, which in turn boosts GH levels in the body. Increased intensity also increases acidity and your body responds by producing the Growth Hormone, a powerful fat loss and muscle building hormone.

CHAPTER TEN: DECIDE HOW LONG TO REST BETWEEN SETS

If you're performing fewer reps, this should mean you're lifting heavier weights and you should be taking longer rests between sets. On the flip side, more reps mean you're lifting lighter weights, so you should have shorter rests between sets. Information collected from various studies, journals and fitness magazines tells us that the optimal amount of rest is **30-90 seconds between each set.**

The idea behind this: More work performed in less time equals an increase in intensity, and increased intensity leads to more muscle growth. You want to do your sets with the least amount of rest between them without risking any type of injury. If you're training for size (hypertrophy) or fitness/conditioning, try to take 30-second rests between your sets. If you're training for power or strength, take up to 90 seconds between sets. However, please use this as a guide and not an absolute. You should listen to your own body and know your own limitations.

Of course, if you're doing any of the three types of supersets, you want to perform the two exercises with no rest in between. However, you can then use the 30-90 second rule for any proceeding sets.

ACTIVE REST

You may have heard the term "active rest," which to me at first seemed like an oxymoron. Active rest allows you to take advantage of the rest period between sets. Therefore, instead of doing nothing but resting, you end up doing a completely different exercise between sets. When implemented properly, active rest allows you to keep working out between sets and makes your workout more efficient and effective. Therefore, you will be able to see the results of your hard work in the gym much sooner.

There are many ways in which active rest can be incorporated into a workout. One example of active rest is: **Skipping for one minute between sets of push-ups**.

Figure 37 Jump Rope / Skipping

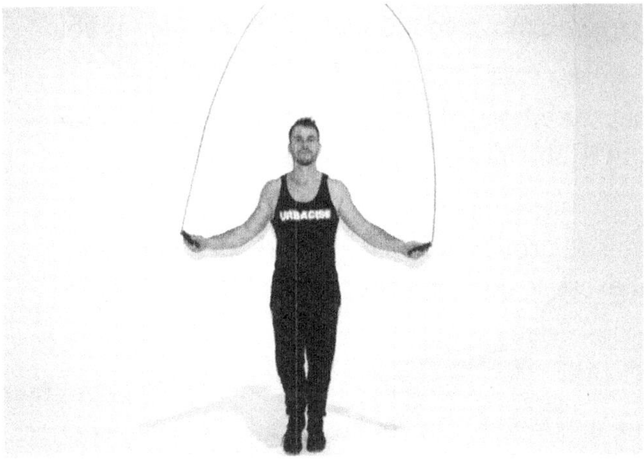

Figure 38: Push-up

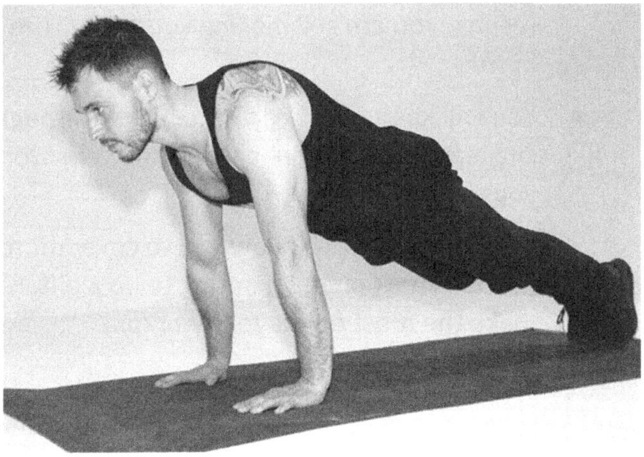

When you do push-ups, you work your chest, arm, and core muscles. Then when you skip between sets of push-ups, you are also working on your cardiovascular fitness and coordination. This, in turn, will help you burn more calories during your workout.

Another example of active rest is: **Jump squats in between sets of bicep curls.**

Figure 39: Jump Squat (Lower)

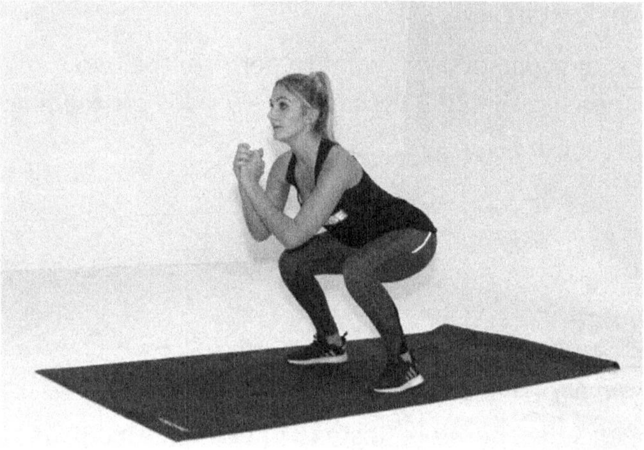

Figure 40: Jump Squat (Upper)

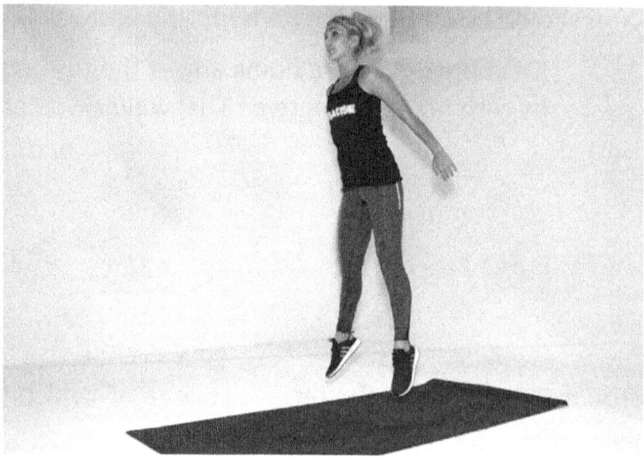

If you do 10-15 jump squats in between sets of bicep curls, you will also end up strengthening and toning your quads, calves, glutes, and hamstrings. Almost any exercise that uses a different muscle group or a different energy system can be done during the "rest" period between sets.

BENEFITS OF ACTIVE REST

- Active rest will help you burn more calories during your workout. This is because instead of resting, you are still moving your body. The more you move your body, the more calories you burn.
- You will keep your heart rate higher throughout the whole workout, which will make it more challenging. The more challenging your workout is, the more progress you will see throughout your fitness journey.
- Active rest will also allow you to cover more muscle groups during your workout. Therefore, if you are short on time, opting to do a different exercise between your sets is the best way to make the most out of your workout.

You will achieve better results if you opt to incorporate active rest into your workouts. Active rest offers a great way to alleviate boredom between sets and is a much better choice than checking your phone as you wait to do your next set. If you are not seeing results from your hard work in the gym, this may be a great way to give your workout a boost.

CHAPTER ELEVEN: HOW MANY EXERCISES PER MUSCLE GROUP

You might be asking yourself how many exercises you should put into your program per muscle group. This will depend on your fitness level, schedule and which split you choose. However, it's recommended that you do between 2 to 6 exercises per muscle group on each of your push, pull and leg days. If we take push day as an example, you'd do 2 to 6 exercises for your chest, 2 to 6 for your shoulders, and 2 to 6 for your triceps.

You could cycle between compound, isolation and machine exercises. This means you can fatigue your muscles even more until you reach failure (either tolerance or tempo failure).

For example, if you were working your shoulders you could do:

- Barbell Military press (Compound)
- Seated Dumbbell Shoulder Press (Compound)
- Dumbbell Front Raise (Isolation)
- Bent-Over Lateral Raise (Isolation)
- Upright Cable Row (Machine)
- Cable Rear-Delt Fly (Machine)

Remember, it's also recommended that you do more pull exercises than push exercises. A lot of people prefer to do chest instead of back, leaving themselves vulnerable to imbalances and injury. Also, remember your scapular is important, so for pull day, it's recommended you do more exercises per muscle group than you would on push day.

If you're using one of the other splits, such as full-body or upper/lower split, then you probably wouldn't be able to perform six exercises per muscle group, as it would take longer, and you would become fatigued.

CHAPTER TWELVE: ADD SOME CARDIO

Cardiovascular exercise is good as it improves the functionality of the body. It can decrease your blood pressure and your resting heart rate so that your heart doesn't have to work as hard. It's also efficient at burning calories, resulting in fat loss. So, it's a good idea to add some cardio to your workout programs.

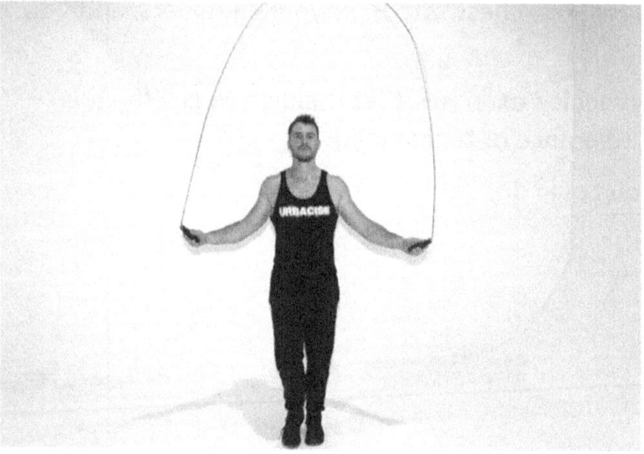

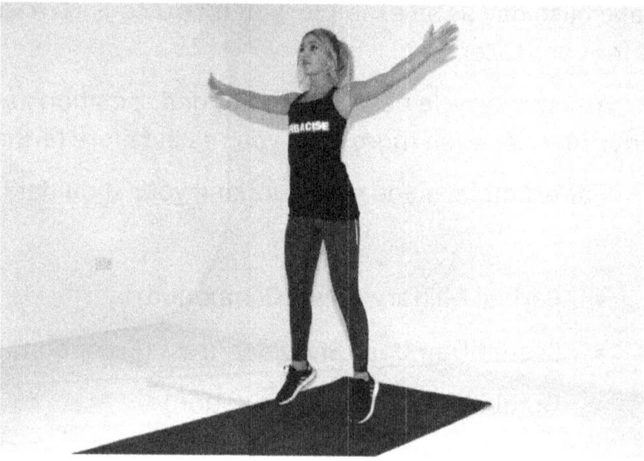

STEADY-STATE CARDIO

Steady-state cardio is where you exercise at a lower intensity - it includes exercises such as running on the treadmill, at a constant speed, or biking at a steady pace.

HIGH-INTENSITY INTERVAL TRAINING (HIIT)

High-Intensity Interval Training (HIIT) isn't aerobic training, but instead anaerobic. This is because HIIT is designed to be done over shorter periods, pushing your limits to their maximum. However, people tend to refer to HIIT as cardio.

HIIT is a type of work out that cycles between short bursts of hard, intense work followed by a short recovery period. This is not to be confused with circuit training, where there is no rest. For example, a person may do as many burpees as they can in 30 seconds, rest for 1 minute, and then repeat that cycle a few times. It's recommended that you do each HIIT exercise for one minute or less. The idea behind HIIT is that you push yourself to your absolute limit, so if you can sustain the exercise longer than one minute, there's a good chance that you are not pushing yourself hard enough. The principle in place here is that we are trying to produce maximum effort to burn fat quicker than we would during a steady-state cardio session: many people say that HIIT training is a good way to get an intense workout in a short period of time.

While HIIT can be done with just about any type of exercise, you need to keep in mind your abilities and limitations. For most ages and experience levels, a stationary bike is best for HIIT training because it is easier on the joints. For athletes, sprints on a track, or uphill, would be a great HIIT workout. This type of training can also be done with weights or bodyweight exercises in the gym or at home.

Doing HIIT workouts enables your body to use energy more efficiently, burning calories (energy) rather than storing calories.

A downside of a HIIT workout is that there is a higher risk of injury if you are new to fitness. Doing too many HIIT workouts in a row can cause burn out. It is recommended to stick to one day of HIIT a week and slowly move up to two days a week from there. How quickly you increase the intensity and number of HIIT workouts is based on your fitness level and the way your body adapts to this type of training.

HIIT can be exhausting, and if you do it too frequently it's easy to over-train. Therefore, it's important to start slowly (if you're new to HIIT training) and gradually increase the intensity over time. This will help to ensure that you have a well-rounded program without over-doing HIIT workouts.

STEADY-STATE VS HIIT

People tend to ask which is better for fat loss: steady-state cardio or HIIT training?

Due to how intense HIIT is, more lactic acid is produced. Your body can use lactic acid as energy, although if you're not able to burn the lactic acid off as quickly as it's created, this will cause a build-up and you won't be able to sustain your workout for as long as steady-state cardio. With HIIT your training sessions are shorter.

During HIIT you are mainly using Adenosine Triphosphate (ATP) to fuel your body. ATP is the energy stored in your muscles. Your body needs to replace any ATP it uses. Over the next 24 - 48 hours, after HIIT, fat is broken down and converted to ATP, so with HIIT you burn more fat after your workout.

To burn the same amount of fat with steady-state cardio, your training sessions must be much longer as they are less intensive. While performing the steady-state cardio, your body begins to use fat as fuel. So, without getting too technical, during a steady-state cardio session (after you have used your primary energy source) you begin to use fat as fuel.

Generally, with steady-state cardio, you begin to burn fat during your workout due to the longer duration, with HIIT you train for a shorter period and burn more fat after the workout.

It's not a question of asking which is better, HIIT or steady-state cardio. Both have their advantages and disadvantages. The question is; what is better for you? If you've been weight training for the last four days, for example, you're probably not going be in a very energetic mood for a HIIT training session, so steady-state may suit you better. Combine both steady-state and HIIT within your exercise program, tweaking it to your fitness level and recovery. However, keep in mind that HIIT is a lot more stimulating and tends to be more effective for fat loss over a shorter training duration.

Here are some additional examples of popular HIIT training routines:

WALK AND SPRINT

- 30-second walk followed by a 30-second sprint
- Repeat this about 8-10 times

As you progress, increase the number of rounds, or do the same routine on a steep gradient.

INFINITE PUSH-UPS

- 10 push-ups at a time. Rest for 30 seconds, and then do 10 more
- To increase the difficulty, rest for 15 seconds instead of 30

You can perform as many rounds as you like.

INFINITE SQUATS

- Perform 10 repetitions, wait 30 seconds, and repeat until you feel the burn

INFINITE BURPEES

- 10 burpees, followed by 30-60 seconds of rest, and then repeat

Stop when you feel exhausted.

The fundamental guidelines we have covered for structuring your workout still apply. However, we suggest that you stick with compound exercises as opposed to isolation exercises, as isolation exercises won't be as effective in a HIIT workout.

CARDIO BEFORE OR AFTER WEIGHTS?

Whether you do cardio before or after lifting weights will depend on your goals. Are you training for any type of endurance-related event? If so, you'd want to put your cardio training first since this is when you will feel the freshest, and you'll be able to push yourself to your maximum effort.

If, however, you are not focused on increasing your endurance or cardio performance, then you'll want to do weight training first. Weight training, like HIIT, is an activity that uses muscle glycogen stores as fuel (ATP). This means that if you deplete these stores with cardio first, you will not be lifting optimally.

Weightlifting can reshape your body and will also increase your metabolism to the greatest extent over the long run. It's recommended that, if you do choose to incorporate cardio within an existing split day, you do your weight training first and do around 15-20 minutes of cardio each session.

In an ideal world, however, you would separate your cardio session from your weightlifting so you can be fresh for both and also reduce the chance of losing muscle mass as you train.

CHAPTER THIRTEEN: WAIT A BIT BEFORE DOING IT AGAIN

The same studies, journals and fitness magazines also help us answer how often we should work out. It's easy to become addicted to how exercise makes us feel. If you're seeing results, sometimes you assume that the more you work out the better your results will be. However, you must remember that the gym is where we tear our muscles. For them to grow back stronger, we need to give them enough time to repair.

It's recommended that you don't work out again for at least 3-5 hours immediately after an intense workout. However, you shouldn't exercise the same muscle group for 48-72 hours afterward. Depending on the split you've chosen, you should wait at least 48 hours before working the same muscle group again.

RECAP

- Full-body split - Wait 48 hours before training again
- Upper/Lower split - Wait 48 hours before working the same muscle groups again. However, you can do the opposing muscle group the next day
- Push/Pull/Legs - Wait 48 hours before working the same muscle group, however, this split offers the greatest freedom over how you want to structure your days

This is a general guide. You know your own body better than anyone else, so listen to it and take as much time to recover as you feel you need.

For more information please see the appendices:

How do muscles grow and recover? (Page 104)

Understand why rest is important (Page 110)

If you over-train and don't give your body enough time to recover (for example by exercising the same muscles less than 48 hours apart), you could begin to feel overly fatigued and your workouts could suffer.

When you first start training, you are probably very motivated, excited and enthusiastic. When you see results, such as an improvement in your fitness level or an increase in strength, you think to yourself "*If a little exercise is good, then more exercise must be better.*" Unfortunately, this is not necessarily true. Sadly, too much exercise, too fast, without adequate rest and recovery, often results in over-training.

Your body will give you physical and mental signs to let you know that you are over-training. Learning to recognize these signs and make the appropriate adjustments will allow you to get your training back on track and avoid more serious complications from over-training.

Signs to be aware of include:

- Changes in your heart rate. If your resting heart rate remains elevated long after your workout ends, your body is telling you it is unable to recover.
- You are constantly tired and sluggish. Over-training uses your supply of glycogen and stored energy beyond your body's ability to replace these stores. Additionally, over-training can deplete your body's hormones resulting in chronic mental and physical fatigue.
- That same hormonal imbalance will cause a lack of motivation, decreased mental alertness and concentration, even a decrease in coordination and ultimately depression.
- Restlessness and an inability to rest, relax or sleep at night. Over-training stresses the body and causes imbalances which upset the normal body functions. That elevated heart rate combined with these imbalances will cause your muscles to twitch and create discomfort in your joints and muscles — all leading to restlessness and the inability to relax.
- You may get sick more often. Over-training will interfere with your immune system, causing you to be more susceptible to colds, flu, respiratory infections and similar illness.
- Loss of appetite. The increased epinephrine and norepinephrine hormone release caused by over-training will result in anxiety and a marked decrease in appetite. Over the long term, this will also result in a decrease in body mass.
- Female trainees may experience menstrual cycle disturbances. Over-training and the resulting imbalances may cause a disruption in a woman's menstrual cycle, including irregular periods or the absence of periods.

Learn to recognize the early symptoms of over-training. Your body needs adequate time to repair, rebuild and recover from the demands that you place on it. To avoid over-training, exercise in moderation and occasionally cut back on your load and intensity.

CHAPTER FIFTEEN: PUSH YOURSELF TO DO MORE (PROGRESSIVE OVERLOAD)

In order to advance in your training program, you need to know about "progressive overload." Our bodies change due to the stress we put them through, so if your body isn't pushed to its limit, then there's no need for it to change/develop. With your training, be it in power, strength, size or fitness, you need to keep making the workouts harder and more intense so that your body doesn't become too comfortable with the exercises you're doing. If you don't change your exercises, you might develop muscle imbalances. You'll also most likely be less motivated and start to think of your training as more of a chore instead of fun.

You can increase the intensity of your program and therefore achieve progressive overload by:

- Adding more weight
- Doing more reps
- Adding more sets
- Training more often
- Taking less rest between sets/exercises

It's recommended that you change your workout program every four to six weeks. This timescale is a rough guide and can change based on your individual goals.

CHAPTER SIXTEEN: RECORD YOUR PROGRESS

There's a famous saying that "**What Gets Measured Gets Improved.**" The only way you can truly tell how well you're progressing in any given exercise program is by recording your results. For example, make a note of the amount of weight you lift each week, and try to increase that weight over the length of your program. Or you can write down the number of reps you achieve in a set amount of time and see if you can beat that number the next time you attempt that exercise.

Hopefully, by making notes on what you achieve in the gym, you'll begin to see a progression. This will give you more confidence, and you'll know that all your hard work is paying off. One of the best ways to record your progress is by writing it down in an exercise log.

For printable exercises logs, login to the download section of the Urbacise.com website:

https://www.urbacise.com/download/

TRAIN HARD – STAY MOTIVATED

We hope you have enjoyed reading this book and have found it both informative and enlightening. You should now have a better understanding of how to structure your exercise programs. Use this new knowledge to improve the efficiency of your work outs and boost your confidence. Plan your training well, and you will no longer wander around the gym, not knowing which exercise to choose next.

If you haven't already, please read all the accompanying appendices, as these cover the topics in more detail and give you an even greater understanding of the body and how it reacts to exercise.

To further help you comprehend the concepts within this book, there are a lot of resources and reference templates available from the download section on Urbacise.com:

https://www.urbacise.com/download/

You can also get advice and ask questions via the community forum, which covers a range of topics from nutrition to the latest exercise equipment:

https://www.urbacise.com/forums/

The best way of learning something is by putting it to use, so if you design an exercise program and would like feedback, you can submit it to Urbacise.com. We'll upload it to our exercise program database where other members can download and try it.

https://www.urbacise.com/upload-exercise-program/

Appendices

Recommended as additional reading

MAJOR MUSCLE GROUPS AND THEIR FUNCTIONS

In any given workout program, you need to do exercises that target each major muscle group. Identifying these muscle groups and what functions they perform is very important because it can help you get in better shape and provide you with a more effective way to improve your fitness.

Our bodies consist of more than 640 muscles that together make up roughly 50% of our bodyweight. Muscles are needed for all vital functions of the body. We use muscles for everything from locomotion to speech, from vision to hearing and from circulating blood to urination — and much more. Living without muscles is impossible. Every muscle or group of muscles is a discrete organ designed to perform a specific function in the body.

Muscles are divided into three different types of tissue based on their structure and anatomical functions. The three types of muscles include Skeletal, Smooth and Cardiac.

1. Skeletal muscles are primarily used to move our bones that are under voluntary control.
2. Smooth muscles are under involuntary control and are found within hollow visceral organs.
3. Cardiac muscles are found within the walls of the heart and are under involuntary control.

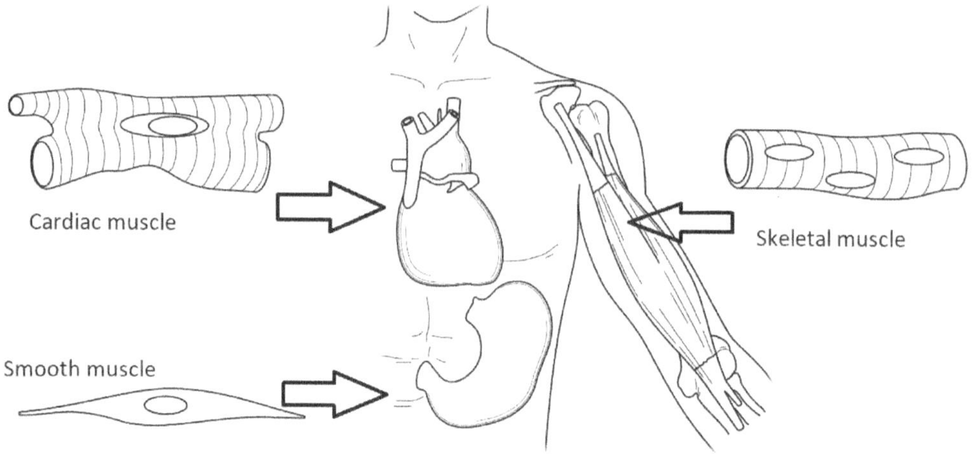

Physiologically, the same type of muscles can perform diverse functions. For example, the biceps and triceps are both skeletal muscles. The biceps are responsible for flexion of the arm while contracting the triceps enable us to extend the arm.

If you've researched muscles before, you're probably familiar with the skeletal muscles. Skeletal muscles are the major players during exercise. However, the functions of the other two types of muscles are also important. All muscles in the body work in harmony. For example, running uses all the muscles of the body:

- Skeletal muscles for moving our arms and legs
- Cardiac muscles to enable the heart to pump extra blood to skeletal muscles
- Smooth muscles in order to dilate the blood vessels in your legs to enable the delivery of oxygenated blood to your legs

When training and developing fitness programs, we concentrate on the skeletal muscles. Below, you will find a brief description of the major skeletal muscles involved in physical activity.

BICEPS AND TRICEPS

These are the front and back muscles of the arm. Biceps enable flexion of the forearm (bending or curling towards your shoulder), while triceps enable an extension of the forearm (moving your forearm away from your shoulder).

ROTATOR CUFF AND DELTOID

These are the major muscles of the shoulder. The deltoid is responsible for the abduction and flexion of the shoulder (lifting and moving the arms). A rotator cuff is a group of four muscles that stabilize the shoulder. When it comes to shoulder movements, they all serve a very important role.

CHEST, CORE AND BACK

The chest is made up of two prominent muscles: the pectoralis major and pectoralis minor. Both muscles enable us to generate force to push objects away from the body. A good example is pushing a heavy door in front of us.

The main muscles of the core include the rectus abdominis (also known as the six-pack muscle) and obliques. Their primary functions are to provide stability to our core as well as enable forward flexion of the spine.

The main back muscles include the latissimus dorsi, teres major, trapezius and rhomboids. All are involved in retraction and pulling — for example, pulling on a rope in a tug of war.

THIGHS AND LEGS

Thighs and legs contain an opposing group of muscles. The quadriceps are the anterior (front) group of thigh muscles. The quadriceps are responsible for extension of the leg. Meanwhile, the hamstrings are the posterior (back) group of muscles. The hamstrings enable us to flex and bend the leg. The tibialis anterior is found on the front of the lower leg. It enables ankle dorsiflexion, which allows us to bring our toes closer to the shin. Meanwhile, on the back of the lower legs, we have gastrocnemius and soleus, which allow us to plantarflex our feet.

HOW DO MUSCLES GROW AND RECOVER?

STRUCTURE OF A MUSCLE

When training, people often concentrate on the visible muscles, which are the skeletal muscles. Very often, we do not focus on our cardiac and smooth muscles. Each skeletal muscle is composed of several muscle fibers.

A muscle fiber is a collection of many muscle cells, known as myocytes. A myocyte is a long, tubular cell that develops from myoblasts to form muscles. The process of forming muscles is known as myogenesis. The sarcoplasm consists of many myofibrils. Myofibrils are long protein cords composed of myofilaments.

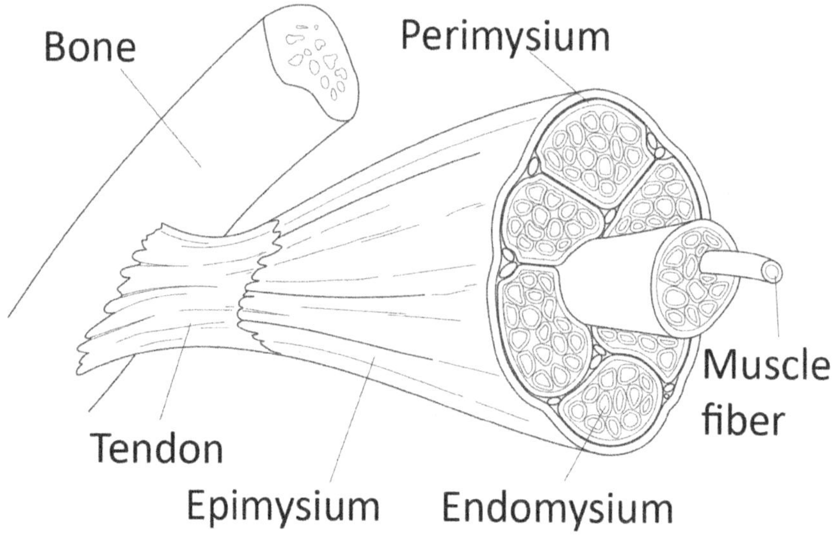

HOW DO MUSCLES GROW AND REPAIR?

Muscle either grows in size or in number. Hypertrophy is when individual muscle fibers grow in size. Hyperplasia is when muscle fibers increase in number. There is another term called "muscular dystrophy," which is a decrease in muscle mass. Muscular dystrophy is often associated with bedridden patients or older people due to a decrease in activity. Whether the body is in the hypertrophic or dystrophic state depends upon your overall health, as well as the quality of your diet and exercise.

Muscular growth, however, depends on several factors including age, gender (men are more muscular than women), hormones (testosterone in men), body adaptations to the exercise demands placed upon it, and genetics. Depending on the nature of your workout, muscle growth is further divided into three phases.

ANABOLIC PHASE

This occurs in the first 40-45 minutes after your workout. During this phase, we often experience muscle pain due to muscle damage. The pain is caused by the accumulation of lactic acid and the breakdown of muscle fibers. Thus, trainers recommend a post-workout protein shake or meat to stimulate muscle recovery. Proper post-workout nutrition will enable you to make gains in muscle strength and endurance.

GROWTH PHASE

In this phase, lactic acid levels drop down to normal, and the body recovers from the damage and replenishes its protein content. It is a period of rapid and sustained muscular growth, which starts after one hour and may last from 5 to 24 hours. An appropriate diet can help the body absorb extra protein, glycogen, and amino acids. All the aforementioned are important nutrients for muscular growth.

REST PHASE

Sleep is a critical time period for the body to repair and recover. Therefore, physicians recommend 8-10 hours of quality sleep. Adequate rest is also necessary for proper muscular growth. Without proper rest, your body will not recover, nor will you be able to reap the full benefits of your workout.

OVERCOMPENSATION CURVE (YAKOVELEV, 1967)

The overcompensation curve shows a phenomenon where resting after a workout causes the body to become stronger and capable of an even greater load. This shows how important rest is, as it will allow you to surpass your previous training efforts.

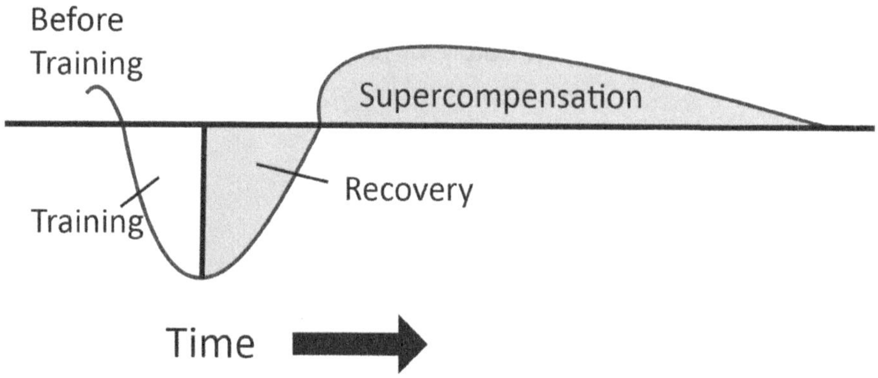

HOW DOES WORKING OUT BUILD MUSCLE?

To fully understand how training and exercise build muscle, you must first understand the musculoskeletal system, muscle fibers, and muscle fiber adaptation. In fitness, as you lift a dumbbell or perform a push-up, the muscles, tendons, joints and supporting bones are under "stress." If you continue to lift that weight or do those push-ups, those muscle fibers, tendons, and supporting structures will "adapt" until your body can perform that exercise without stress.

Therefore, when we train, we are effectively damaging our muscles causing tiny tears, also called "micro-tears," in our muscle fibers. You have probably woken up the day after exercise and been sore. This is known as Delayed Onset Muscle Soreness (DOMS), which is where you're feeling the effects that these micro-tears have on your body.

Then our bodies begin to repair themselves, aided through rest and our diet. Our muscles repair themselves in order to get stronger and more efficient at dealing with the stress caused by workouts. Therefore, our bodies adapt to stress, exercise or movement. In other words, this could be seen as an evolutionary defense. Since we are not strong enough to deal with our environment, we adapt in order to give ourselves the best chance of survival.

Once your body has adapted to the stress of your current workout, you will not get any stronger until you understand the progressive overload principle. Without progressively overloading your muscles, your body will feel like it no longer needs to adapt. Therefore, you will never get bigger or stronger beyond this stage. You must gradually force your muscles to do more for them to grow and get stronger.

DENSE MUSCLE VS. BIG MUSCLE

Previously, we spoke about how muscle either grows in size or in number. Muscular strength is not strictly dependent on muscle size. Some people are compact and strong primarily because their muscles are dense, which means they have more muscle fibers. On the other hand, some people are larger despite their muscles being less dense. This physiological difference is best demonstrated by two very different types of weightlifters you might run into at the gym.

BODYBUILDERS AND POWERLIFTERS

Bodybuilders and powerlifters both train hard and use pretty much the same equipment, however, they have very different training goals and objectives. The powerlifter trains strictly for strength while the bodybuilder trains for size and appearance.

POWERLIFTERS

With few exceptions, powerlifters are not as big or muscular as bodybuilders. They primarily train for strength and always strive to lift more weight. This strength training develops strong, dense muscles that allow them to bench press, squat and deadlift more weight than bodybuilders can even dream of lifting. Powerlifters train and compete using low reps and explosive power. This type of training causes muscle hypertrophy and an increase in strength.

BODYBUILDERS

Bodybuilders, on the other hand, often train with lighter weights at higher reps, usually with a smooth, even cadence. They train for volume and "the pump." This results in sarcoplasmic hypertrophy, which is an increase in sarcoplasmic fluid.

If you prefer to be lean with dense, strong muscles, then concentrate on doing fewer sets with heavy weights and do less than 5 reps per set.

However, if you prefer to be bigger and more muscular for the sake of appearance, do sets of 8-12 reps or more using lighter weights, but not too light.

FREE WEIGHTS OR MACHINES?

Which are better, free weights or machines? Choosing one over the other would depend on your goals as well as your knowledge of your own biomechanics, in terms of proper exercise form. You would also want to know the difference between isolation and compound exercises. Both machines and free weights can serve a very different purpose and play an important role when developing an exercise program.

BENEFITS OF EXERCISE MACHINES:

- **Machines are safer to use** – If you are new to the gym, a lot of exercise injuries happen due to people lifting too heavy a weight with bad biomechanics (bad biomechanics is also referred to as having "bad form" when performing an exercise). An example of bad form would be not keeping your back straight while performing a barbell squat or leaning too far forward, and this could result in serious back injury. However, using a machine restricts your bodies movements and therefore makes you less susceptible to injury.
- **They can help you combat imbalances** – Our bodies are made up of opposing muscle groups, which basically means we have a "front" and "back" muscle stretching over each of our joints. A popular example in your arm would be your bicep (front muscle) and tricep (back muscle). If you are not following a very good exercise program, resulting in your triceps becoming overdeveloped, you could "isolate" your bicep with a bicep curl machine. This would ensure you work your bicep as efficiently as possible without affecting your triceps as much as you would if you were using free weights.
- **Proportionality bigger body part** – Because machines allow us to better isolate our body parts, it's easier to develop individual muscles. This would be for the sake of aesthetics, such as bodybuilding., Some people want a bigger chest, biceps or glutes. Machines can help develop these body parts to achieve the desired result.
- **Good for overloading individual muscles when you can no longer perform heavy compound exercises** – It's recommended when doing a workout, you start by exercising the biggest muscles first (performing compound exercises). After a while, your muscles will become fatigued. Machines, particularly those machines that are isolation exercises, are a good way to push your muscles further

DRAWBACKS OF EXERCISE MACHINES:

- **Not great for full body development** – With machines mainly being isolation exercises, it is therefore not advisable to only perform machine exercises in your workout plan. A healthy way of looking at exercise is to try and keep your body as balanced as possible in terms of muscle development.

- **Machines are "guiding"** – Meaning they dictate how you move your body, so they don't help develop stabilizer muscles (also known as secondary or synergist muscles). So, if machine exercises are not put into a well-balanced exercise program, they can often result in an increased risk of poor posture or chronic injury.
- **Machines can give you a false sense of security** – Due to the simplicity of machine exercises they can pose a risk of direct or indirect injury if, for example, they feel too safe or easy to use.
- **Machines are expensive, fixed locally and require more room** – They're not cost-effective compared to a barbell or set of dumbbells, so if you're looking for a home workout machines, they may not be the best option.

BENEFITS OF FREE WEIGHTS:

- **Free weights allow you to move more naturally** – This means you tend to engage your stabilizer muscles more. This is true especially in full-body compound exercises (meaning exercises involving more than one joint) such as a clean and press. When performed with the correct form, free weight exercises can help develop better posture.
- **Free weights allow for a better Range of Motion (ROM)** – Hence providing greater carryover to your daily activities. Dumbbells are good for developing good ROM. For example, dumbbell bench press allows you to go "deeper" in the lower phase of the exercise than you'd be able to go with a barbell.
- **Compared to machines, free-weights provide endless variations** – For example, you could combine weighted squats and military press, forming a superset, exercising different muscle groups together (legs and shoulders). Other variations can include carrying, pressing, squatting, and swinging.
- **They are less bulky and cheaper** – Working out from home with free weights can be achieved for very little cost., You can easily store them to one side until they're needed.

DRAWBACKS OF FREE WEIGHTS:

- **Without knowledge of proper technique, it's easy to get injured** - It's recommended that if you don't know how to perform an exercise, check out our exercise database for a detailed tutorial.
- **Sometimes dependent on other people's help** – Heavy free-weight exercises such as the barbell bench press often require the help of a spotter (a person to support your heavier lifts).
- **Imbalances if performed incorrectly** – Slight differences in the weight or using the wrong technique can result in an imbalanced physique.

Generally, free weight exercises focus on total body strength and compound movements, while machines are good tools for targeting specific muscle groups through isolation exercises. When looking at the benefits and drawbacks of machines vs free weights, the choice of which one to use depends on you and your goal. Ideally, you should combine both into your workouts, developing a well-designed and balanced exercise program that will allow you to meet your dream physique, level of fitness or level of strength.

UNDERSTANDING WHY REST IS IMPORTANT

Moderate aerobic exercises like walking, cycling, and climbing stairs need much less rest between intervals, especially when you are not concerned with weight training or reshaping your body. This rule applies to low to moderate workout intensities. However, if you are training at high intensities or are new to weightlifting and you get sore after every workout (DOMS), you should be resting more in order to stimulate muscle recovery. Therefore, in order to determine how long you should rest between workouts, it is necessary to find out why rest is so important between workouts and what happens when you don't take the time to recover.

PHYSIOLOGY OF REST AND MUSCLE GROWTH

The amount of rest is just as important as the number of reps. The goal of your workout should be to overload your muscles, which will eventually result in exhaustion and fatigue. As we know, heavy weights cause minor tears in your muscles. This is all part of the process and should not be confused with tears caused by traumatic injuries. This breakdown of muscle fibers (proteins) is required for muscle growth. Although the outcome of training is minor muscle breakdown, adequate rest and recovery enable your muscles to heal and rebuild.

HOW LONG SHOULD I REST BETWEEN WORKOUTS?

The answer to this question largely depends on your workout routine, specific goal and your personal preferences. The rule of thumb is that you should rest enough to allow your muscles to fully recover.

The following factors determine how long you need to rest between your workouts:

- **Frequency** – How often you exercise per day and per week.
- **Intensity** – In the world of training, this means how hard you hit the gym or how challenging your workout was.

- **Nutrition** – What type of food you eat, how much food you eat, when you eat, and how often you eat can determine your recovery requirements.
- **Duration** - This includes the time you are performing the specific exercise (for example: how many reps and sets of bicep curls you do in a workout).

All the aforementioned factors vary widely among individuals. The need for recovery depends upon an individual's fitness level, time spent at the gym, diet, daily routine, as well as their body's ability to handle the challenging workouts.

Resting times are divided into three categories:

- Between sets of an exercise (Seconds)
- Immediately following exercise (Hours)
- Between the exercise of one group of muscles (Days)

Information collected from various studies, journals and fitness magazines shows the following resting guidelines:

- 30-90 seconds rest between sets
- 3-5 hours immediately after an intense workout
- 48-72 hours after exercise of specific groups of muscles (for example, if you did legs on Monday, then you should not do legs again until Wednesday or Thursday)

When it comes to exercise, more is not always better. Therefore, schedule your workouts in a way that allows you to recover properly. Follow the guidelines above and you will get the most out of your exercise routine.

SHOULD I STRETCH BEFORE OR AFTER MY WORKOUT?

Stretching is an important part of maintaining your overall fitness and keeping yourself limber and flexible. We have been told for years that stretching is an essential part of a fitness program to make sure that the body is properly prepared for physical activity. However, what type of stretching should we practice? When is the best time to stretch, before or after a workout? Are there any real benefits to stretching?

WHAT HAPPENS WHEN YOU STRETCH?

Cats know that it's not their paws that help them climb safely over walls or jump over obstacles, but rather their great flexibility. But where does this flexibility come from?

A muscle fiber, as we know now, is composed of several sarcomeres (the basic unit of contraction in the muscle fiber) connected together. In turn, many muscle fibers join to make a whole muscle. In a normal state, these muscle fibers are closely packed with each other and are disorganized. Stretching tends to deliberately contract or flex the muscle in such a way that it lengthens. It also helps the body to realign any disorganized fibers in the direction of the tension. Stretched muscles are thus more flexible and pliable.

WHAT TYPE OF STRETCHING IS THE BEST?

There are two basic types of stretches: static and dynamic. Static stretching is usually held for 20-30 seconds or more in the same position (think of touching your toes while standing). Recommendations as to whether you should be doing static stretches vary from year to year and expert to expert. Some people believe it hinders physical performance. At the same time, others tend to think that it has its own benefits, such as improved flexibility and posture.

On the other hand, dynamic or PNF (Proprioceptive Neuromuscular Facilitation) stretching involves active movements that tend to resemble an actual workout or sport-specific moves, such as walking lunges, butt kicks, and hip circles.

The active motion during a dynamic stretch helps maintain your body at a higher core temperature. Research indicates that dynamic stretching improves your muscle strength, anaerobic capacity, agility, and overall performance. Additionally, some even claim that it is a safe and more effective way to prepare your body for the activity to come.

Static stretching is most beneficial during the cool down phase. After a training session, the muscles are more pliable. However, dynamic stretching before any workout will minimize the chances of injury and is better suited for preparing your body for a workout.

IS DELAYED ONSET MUSCLE SORENESS (DOMS) GOOD OR BAD?

You have probably experienced burning pain in your legs, shoulders or other parts of the body after a tough workout. This post-exercise soreness in the muscles is called Delayed Onset Muscle Soreness (DOMS). It usually develops 6-8 hours after exercise and reaches its peak intensity after 48-72 hours. DOMS is characterized by mild pain, muscle soreness or burning sensations. Although it tends to be more common in the lower region, it can affect any muscle group in the body that has recently been through extensive stretching or an intense gym session.

WHAT CAUSES DOMS?

People once thought DOMS was caused by the accumulation of lactic acid and degenerative metabolic products. This theory has been disproven by a research paper published by Bard Schoenfeld and Bret Contreras. The article suggests the underlying cause of DOMS is the activation and stimulation of nociceptors (pain receptors) followed by acute inflammation. The inflammation stems from microscopic tears in the muscle. These tears stimulate the pain receptors, heightening the sensations of pain. Therefore, tiny tears in the muscle fibers are responsible for DOMS.

IS DOMS GOOD OR BAD?

DOMS is soreness or pain related to muscles, tendons or ligaments. Any pain felt in the joints or the bones do not fall under the umbrella of DOMS. Joint pain is always bad. Sharp pains or bolts of pain indicate a severe muscle injury or a significant trauma. DOMS comes hours after a workout and is relatively mild.

The famous phrase "no pain, no gain," is often associated with a job well done, and although it is catchy, it isn't necessarily true. There has been no scientific research that proves DOMS is directly proportional to muscular hypertrophy (an increase in the size of the muscle). Some people have achieved muscular growth and an athletic look without ever experiencing any soreness. DOMS varies from person to person and may have some genetic predisposition, so don't despair if you don't get sore after exercise.

You'll be more likely to develop DOMS if you don't prepare your body for exercise, so always warm up before starting any exercise. Remember to stay well hydrated and don't neglect your cardio training, as it helps your body become more efficient and healthier.

THE IMPORTANCE OF REFUELING AFTER A WORKOUT

Known as nutrient timing, what you eat before, during, and after your workouts is extremely important in order to maximize your results. Whether you are trying to lose weight, build muscle or train for a specific sport, you need to feed your body the right nutrients in the right amounts at the right time. What you eat beforehand prepares your body for your workout. What you take in after your workout maximizes the benefits you will get from your exercise session while preparing your body for the next workout.

Most experts agree that nutrition is even more important than the workout itself. Our bodies need to repair and recover from the intensity of the workouts. Your muscles will be craving glycogen, electrolytes and water. Glycogen fuels your muscle cells and is transported to the muscles with water. Therefore, you need to make sure you hydrate and add some electrolytes to your diet.

Your post-workout meal is the one that plays the largest role in supplying your body with everything that it will need to repair, rebuild, recover, as well as adapt to the beating that you have given your muscles during your workout. You must provide your muscles with what they need to recover and grow. A efficient workout is not complete until you properly refuel.

There are five main food groups, and the first three are the most beneficial when refueling after a workout:

- **Carbohydrates** – for energy
- **Fats** – for stored energy (and extreme sports)
- **Protein** – for growth, maintenance, and repair
- **Milk and dairy products**
- **Fruit and vegetables**

BENEFITS OF REFUELING AFTER A HEAVY WORKOUT

PREVENTS MUSCLE BREAKDOWN

A tough strength training workout will create microscopic tears in your muscle fibers. If adequate nutrients are not supplied before and/or after the workout, these muscle tears can lead to further muscle breakdown. This means that your muscle will be broken down to form protein that your body uses as energy to repair itself.

INCREASES PROTEIN SYNTHESIS

After a strenuous workout, your body is biochemically primed to absorb nutrients. Your muscles are highly insulin-sensitive, which means that the carbs you eat help muscle recovery, instead of getting converted into fat. Insulin is a storage hormone that has a bad reputation because it is integral to fat gain. After a workout, however, insulin is your friend, and a proper post-workout meal can help you build muscle and lose fat.

FASTER RECOVERY

A properly timed post-workout meal with the right nutrients can help decrease soreness in your muscles after a challenging workout. For example, if you are able to recover in only a day as opposed to 2-3 days, that means you can train harder and more frequently, which will lead to better and faster results.

GLYCOGEN REPLENISHMENT

Regardless of the type of workout, if you are working out intensely, your body will use glycogen as fuel. Glycogen, which is stored in your muscles and liver, is best described as your body's preferred fuel source for workouts. Depending on the duration, type, and intensity of exercise, glycogen stores can become depleted. Eating ample carbs after a workout can not only promote protein synthesis, but also help replenish energy stores to keep you feeling energetic for the rest of the day.

FOODS THAT ARE BEST FOR REFUELING

- Sandwich Wraps
- Sweet Potatoes
- Whole-grain Breakfast Cereal
- Eggs

In life and in fitness, consistency is one of the main secrets to success. You cannot workout occasionally and expect to see real results. This also holds true when it comes to your post-workout nutrition. We all know that consistency over time will bring about major changes. Feed your muscles what they need before and after every workout and you will be amazed at the body you will achieve.

GLOSSARY

1 Rep Max – One rep maximum or 1RM is the maximum amount of weight a person can lift if attempting to lift a load only once.

Active Rest - Active rest allows you to take advantage of the rest period between sets by doing a completely different exercise between sets.

Aerobic - Also known as cardio, whereby you exercise to strengthen your heart, lungs, and improve your body's overall efficiency in using oxygen.

Agonist - The muscle that moves whilst performing an exercise.

Anabolic phase - The first 40-45 minutes after your workout.

Anaerobic - Mainly weightlifting type exercises designed to improve strength, speed and power and popular with bodybuilders and powerlifters.

Antagonistic - A muscle that opposes the agonist muscle.

Barbell - The long metal bar you find in the gym that you can add weights to and use for bodybuilding, powerlifting, and general fitness.

Bodybuilder – A person who increases the size of their muscles by lifting heavy things, such as weights.

Cardiac muscles - Found within the walls of the heart and under involuntary control.

Circuit Training - Where you complete several different exercises in quick succession with minimal rest.

DOMs - Delayed Onset Muscle Soreness.

Dumbbell - A smaller metal bar with weight often fixed on, designed to be used one-handed in pairs of two.

Drop Sets - Drop sets allow you to extend your set in order to increase muscle fibers and fatigue the muscle as much as possible, training until failure.

Duration - This includes the time you are performing the specific exercise (for example: how many reps and sets of bicep curls you do in a given workout).

Dynamic Stretching - Stretches that mimic your actual workout, such as bodyweight lunges, squats and high knees.

Failure - There are three types of failure: tempo, technique and tolerance. Technique failure is the one that causes injury when people perform the exercise with incorrect form.

Flexibility - Improves the range of motion of your joints allowing your joints to move freely and improve the overall mobility of your muscles.

Free Weights - Equipment that is not attached, including barbells and dumbbells.

Frequency – How often you exercise per day and per week.

Growth phase - From 5 to 24 hours after a workout. In this phase, lactic acid levels drop down to normal, the body recovers from the damage and replenishes its protein content.

HIIT - High-Intensity Interval Training, a type of workout that cycles between short bursts of hard, intense work followed by a short recovery period.

Hyperplasia - When muscle fibers increase in number.

Hypertrophy - When individual muscle fibers grow in size.

Intensity – In the world of training, it means how hard you hit the gym or how challenging your workout was.

Lactic Acid – A byproduct of anaerobic glycolysis, found in the muscle tissue.

Machines - Equipment consisting of pulleys, wires, pins and weight stacks that are usually fixed to one point.

Micro-tears - Small tears in the muscle fibers caused by working out. The body repairs these and adapts the muscle fibers to be stronger.

Muscle fibers - These are the cells that make up the skeletal muscles.

Nutrition – What type of food you eat, how much food you eat, when you eat, and how often you eat. This can determine your recovery requirements.

Powerlifters - A person who increases the density of their muscles by lifting heavy things, such as weights. Normally concentrating on explosive power.

Progressive overload - The principle whereby the body changes due to increased increase in volume, intensity, frequency or time. If your body isn't pushed to its limit, then there's no need for it to change/develop.

Pyramid Sets - Pyramid sets give you the chance to gradually warm up as you raise the intensity of your exercise.

Range of Motion (ROM) - The movement potential of a joint.

Rep - Repetitions are simply the number of times you perform an exercise, abbreviated in the gym to reps. For example, if you do two push-ups, that means you've effectively done two reps of push-ups.

Rotator Cuff - A rotator cuff is a group of four muscles that stabilize the shoulder.

Scapular - Also known as the shoulder blade, the scapular is responsible for the movement of the shoulder.

Set - A set is the number of cycles you do of a particular exercise. If I did 20 push-ups, 20 is the number of reps. If I then choose to do that three times, I would be doing three sets of push-ups, doing 20 reps each time.

Skeletal muscle - Primary function is to move our bones, which are under voluntary control.

Smooth muscles - Under involuntary control and are found within hollow visceral organs.

Split - A split is where you divide your workouts by muscle group., The most popular splits are full-body, upper/lower and push/pull/legs.

Spotter - A person who watches you lift weight in case you get in trouble, and to help prevent injury.

Stability - Without the correct alignment of your joints, you use your muscles to try and compensate for poor stability.

Staggered sets - Staggered sets train completely unrelated muscle groups.

Static Stretching - Where you hold the stretch for a certain amount of time. Touching your toes for 30 seconds is an example.

Steady-State Cardio - Where you exercise for prolonged periods of time at a lower intensity (such as running or cycling).

Straight Sets - Straight sets are the most common sort of set and are simply where you do as many reps as you can, rest in between sets in order to let your body recover, and then do the same amount of sets (with the same amount of weight) again.

Supersets - A superset is performed by combining two exercises back to back with no rest in between.

Synergist - Smaller supporting muscles.

Made in the USA
Middletown, DE
20 March 2023

27171465R00066